GENEFIT NUTRITION®

Genefit Nutrition®

Nutrition Designed by Life

ROMAN DEVIVO
&
ANTJE SPORS

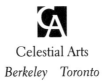

Celestial Arts

Berkeley   Toronto

Distributed in Australia by Simon & Schuster Australia, in Canada by Ten Speed Press Canada, in New Zealand by Southern Publishers Group, in South Africa by Real Books, in Southeast Asia by Berkeley Books, and in the United Kingdom and Europe by Airlift Book Company.

Library of Congress Cataloging-in-Publication Data

Devivo, Roman, 1967–
  Genefit nutrition : nutrition by life / by Roman Devivo and Antje Spors.
    p. cm.
  ISBN 1-58761-163-5 (alk. paper)
  1. Nutrition. 2. Instinct. 3. Food habits. I. Spors, Antje, 1972– .II. Title.
RA784 .D49 2003
613.3—dc21   2002152236

1   2   3   4   —   05   04   03

Printed in the U.S.A.

— CONTENTS —

Foreword   vii

Acknowledgments   ix

Introduction   xi

PART ONE
Theoretical Foundations

1. Genefit Nutrition: An Overview   3
2. A Question of Adaptation   13
3. The Human Nutritional Instinct   34

PART TWO
Rediscover Your Nutritional Instinct

4. Eating Pleasure as Guide   41
5. The Instinctively Balanced Diet   51
6. What Is a "Natural" Food?   62
7. The Nose Knows   87
8. The Question that Drives Us   97

9. Peace of Mind   104

10. Foods that Poison and Symptoms that Heal   111

PART THREE
Do It Yourself

11. Before You Jump   137

12. Welcome to the Guidelines of Genefit Nutrition   143

13. The Other Half of Success—Your Toolbox   152

14. Food Supply: Processing Techniques   158
    and Treatments

15. Food Groups and Meal Sequences   164

16. What to Expect   177

PART FOUR
Food, Health, and Illness

17. Food and Allergies   187

18. Food and Cancer   192

19. Food and Autoimmune Diseases   198

20. Food and Weight Management   203

21. Food and Cardiovascular Diseases   205

22. Food and Diabetes   207

23. Food and Viruses   210

24. Food and the Practice of Medicine   218

PART FIVE
Genefit Nutrition: Present and Future

25. Testimonials   225

26. Genefit Nutrition: A Vision of the Future   230

    Appendices   235

By Harvey Diamond,
co-author of *Fit for Life*

FOR CENTURIES, the quest for the ideal diet has caused much ink to flow. Many of us have already addressed, and will continue to address, this simple and basic question: How and what should we eat to guarantee our children and ourselves a long and healthy life? Over the past century, a number of medical discoveries have clearly demonstrated the impact dietary habits can have on our health. As a consequence the awareness of the importance of a healthy diet has tremendously increased in the past fifty years. But how do we define a healthy diet? Once we try to answer this question we unavoidably generate thousands of new ones. According to the concept of Genefit Nutrition, out of all those questions, ironically, only one might lead to the actual answer: "To what kind of diet are we genetically adapted?" Is it really that simple? For what type of fuel has our biological engine been built? Well, it seems that the answer lies in our genes, and therefore in our evolutionary past.

The twenty-first century is the century of the genes — the century when we are coming to understand the code of life. As history has shown, scientific knowledge can bring the best and, unfortunately, also the worst. The power to genetically modify organisms makes the hypothesis of a possible mismatch between our genes and modern food more crucial than ever.

There aren't many researchers who have looked closely at nutrition in the context of genetics and evolution. Even among the hundreds of thousands of researchers, nutritionists, and dieticians all over the world, the fundamental question of genetic adaptation to food is too rarely taken into consideration.

In bringing together fields such as genetics, anthropology, chemistry, molecular biology, medicine, and nutritional sciences, this book, based on decades of empirical research, constitutes an outstanding piece of work. *Genefit Nutrition: Nutrition Designed by Life* will not only provide a solid theoretical background, but also a series of simple experiments you can easily perform for yourself to demonstrate the empirical foundations of the concept.

I decided to write the foreword for this revolutionary book because it seemed to me that it sets forth the concept of a truly natural diet in a much more fundamental way than most approaches I've seen before. If you are ready, beyond all prejudices, to reconsider what is on your daily kitchen table, this book definitely is for you. Some will adore it, others might hate it, but I can assure you it won't leave you indifferent.

Enjoy the ride.

—*Harvey Diamond*

— ACKNOWLEDGMENTS —

THIS BOOK is the result of amazing teamwork. Over the past four decades, numerous people have been involved in the development of Genefit Nutrition, from those who simply practiced it to those who studied the physiological and psychological mechanisms underlying this wonderful way of eating. Every one of them brought a little piece to the puzzle. Throughout the history of Genefit Nutrition, contributions have been made at many different levels: scientific, medical, financial, and personal. If this book should be dedicated to someone, it is our deepest wish to dedicate it to all those involved in the process of making Genefit Nutrition what it has become.

Our special thanks go to Helen Young and the now deceased Severen Schaeffer for putting ideas and concepts into words in a much better way than we could ever have done.

—*Roman Devivo and Angtje Spors*, LOS ANGELES, 2002

FOR US PROUDLY CIVILIZED HUMANS, the principles at the origin of Genefit Nutrition are almost four decades old, but if we adopt the viewpoint of the other eighty million species who share our planet, Genefit Nutrition is not less than three billion years old. It is the natural diet practiced by every animal on earth, even though there are some variations depending on species. In nature, optimal health is essential for survival, yet no living being except modern humans ever needed dietetic knowledge to stay healthy. Throughout the history of life, high-quality nutrients contained in food provided directly by nature and an infallible instinctual dietary guidance have always been the best guarantees for health and top fitness. The need for dietetic research for us to get healthy is in itself an indication that we have lost something along our evolutionary path. Genefit Nutrition is the way to get it back.

This extraordinary way of eating has been regularly updated to incorporate the most recent findings in nutritional research, dietetics, and nutritional anthropology. Decades of continuous observations on a wide array of people have slowly and steadily brought Genefit Nutrition to its current, robust state. Besides being ultimately natural, Genefit Nutrition, for the first time in dietetic history, utilizes the built-in nutritional instinct each one of us possesses as the best guide to optimal health and dietary balance.

Genefit Nutrition can either be applied for a limited period of time or span a lifetime. The choice is yours: If your current lifestyle doesn't allow you to apply Genefit Nutrition all the time, it is still enormously beneficial to take advantage of its powerful positive effects over short periods of three days, three weeks, or even once or twice a year. Your body will always profit from the cleansing processes triggered by contact with completely natural foods. For example, a 21-day cleanse will help you lose unnecessary pounds and rid the body of various toxins and harmful molecules that are unavoidable in a diet of traditional processed food. Detoxification is the best method for preventing serious pathologies; in addition, Genefit Nutrition replenishes the nutritional deficiencies caused by the process of cooking and preserving foods.

If your current life conditions allow you to apply Genefit for a longer period of time, you will experience the extraordinary physiological and psychological state one can be in when the body and brain return to their original state of functioning. After a short adjustment period, your body will demonstrate new abilities and characteristics you never thought possible. The absence of abnormal artificial molecules in the bloodstream and brain will, among many other benefits, give you an unprecedented inner quietness and a permanent relaxation of the nervous system.

Rediscovering your own nutritional instinct is probably the most exciting part of all. You won't need to worry about what to eat and what not to eat to obtain better health. The nutritional instinct will engender self-confidence and trust in your own body, along with a way of eating full of fun and pleasure. It is also a symbol of freedom and independence: no more relying on the food industry, which has shown itself to produce unhealthy food for the sake of profit, and no more relying on ever-changing dietary trends, which are unable to answer the most vital questions. With Genefit Nutrition, you will feel in control of your own life and your own body, because you will be able to find the answers within yourself.

In this book we will not tell you that a diet rich in protein or a diet low in calories is best for your health or your figure. We will not tell you what you should eat on Mondays and what you shouldn't eat on Thursdays, because we honestly don't know. Anybody who tells you otherwise isn't telling you the truth. It is impossible for anybody to know exactly what you should eat, or how much you should eat to achieve dietary balance and optimal health. Each individual has different needs, depending on both internal and external factors, and those needs vary from day to day. Therefore, dietary advice and prescription can never be really accurate; they will never fit your particular needs precisely. No one but you can determine what your body really needs at a given moment. For all these reasons, we do not provide any recipe or prescription as far as the actual diet is concerned. All we do is explain how to set up the right conditions for your nutritional instinct to work and teach you how to listen and interpret your own sensory and bodily signals so that three billion years of life experience will take over. No prescription diet can compete with that.

—*Roman Devivo and Antje Spors*

DISCLAIMER — READER PLEASE NOTE

The recommendations in this book are not intended as medical advice. Before undertaking the practice of Genefit Nutrition, particularly if you are under medical supervision or are taking medication for a specific physical problem, you are advised to consult with your physician.

If you decide to take up eating by instinct and find it isn't working for you, then stop. The intent of this book is to point out things you may do, not things you must do. The book explains that food can constitute a potent therapeutic tool, but this observation should not be construed as an incitement to abandon medical treatment. Particularly with respect to medical drugs, before making any changes, consult with the physician who prescribed them. It must be understood that a book cannot substitute for the help a beginner might need to recognize toxin-laden foods and properly select unprocessed foods for effectiveness. For this reason, although the authors have made every effort to provide the most accurate information, they cannot assume responsibility for any interpretation and use the reader may make of it.

— PART ONE —

Theoretical Foundations

ONE

Genefit Nutrition:
An Overview

Ironically, our greatest achievement as a species may be applying
our enlarged brain and our technology to recreating the diet we
instinctively ate a million years ago.

—TVA Newsletter, November–December 1996

MOST PEOPLE TODAY are aware that nutrition plays a vital role in
their health. You are probably concerned with eating a "balanced" diet
containing sufficient minerals, vitamins, fibers, etc. You are also probably a bit confused as to just exactly what "sufficient" might mean. At various times you may have tried one diet or another, one type of food supplement or another, one or another nutritional philosophy. The chances
are that for a time, or to a degree, whatever you were doing made you
feel more vital, or lose some weight. And then, for some reason, it
stopped working, or it became difficult or unsatisfying to continue. Then
you just forgot about dieting or skipped taking supplements for a while,
until a new diet or formula caught your attention.

Or maybe at some point you adopted a nutritional system such as
macrobiotics, for instance, and decided that this was "The Way," once
and for all. In order to fully benefit from Genefit Nutrition, we would
like to invite you to momentarily put aside your beliefs and attend to
your senses, which will then guide you more accurately than dietary precepts could ever do.

In a sense, we are what we eat. Food can make us healthy, but it can
also make us both physiologically and psychologically ill, and it can even
kill us. Ironically, much of what we generally consume in our quest for
the former is actually doing the latter. Usually it does so slowly so we

often fail to recognize it. On the other hand, food can also give us health and vitality. In the following chapters, we will describe a method for preventing and healing minor as well as major health problems. We will explain how to achieve well being and a higher quality of life with foods selected by instinct. Since its discovery, this method has even been shown to generate recoveries in conditions that are normally considered incurable.

Genefit Nutrition is based on the discovery that humans are as fully endowed as animals with a genetically determined nutritional instinct, and that this built-in programming can guide us to the food that will keep us well and support health and recovery. It teaches us to use our senses to choose the nutrients our bodies truly need, free from restrictive precepts or recipes. Genefit Nutrition is neither a diet nor a system. Instead, it the most natural way of eating there is, especially because it is based exclusively on unprocessed food. Here, however, "unprocessed" should be understood as synonymous with "original," or literally food that is in the state in which it is found in nature. A food that has been ground, frozen, cooked, mixed, seasoned, or otherwise "denatured" in any way, even slightly, does not fit the very precise food quality requirements of Genefit Nutrition. Fruits or vegetables bred by artificial selection and/or grown on chemical fertilizers, and animals fed hormones, mixed grains, etc., are not strictly unprocessed according to this definition. The food supply Genefit Nutrition demands must be as natural as it can be.

Genefit Nutrition is the result of an unprecedented study — a study of what happens when humans and animals exclusively consume foods in their original, unmodified state, selecting them by instinctive sense-cues alone. It differs substantially from the nutritional philosophy of "raw-foodism" that already existed at the time of Socrates, and has become once again popular today. The idea that "raw food is good for us" is correct as far as it goes, but is incomplete and sometimes even dangerous without instinctive intake regulation.

The fundamentals of Genefit Nutrition originated from the evolution of life on earth. According to the latest development in science, the fossil record indicates that the simplest life forms appeared on earth roughly 3 billion years ago, and that their evolution into cellular and then multicellular organisms was very slow. Here and there mutations occurred, which started new lineages leading to plankton, fish, lizards, birds, and insects. Small mammals first appeared approximately a hundred million years ago. As they evolved along divergent developmental lines, they gave rise to monkeys and apes some sixty-five million years ago, and finally to our first human ancestors, who appeared about six million years ago. Man's earliest use of fire dates back roughly 400,000 years; agriculture, the consumption of wheat and other grains, and animal husbandry began only around 8,000 B.C.

If we were to imagine the course of life evolution as a road twenty-five miles long, humans would come into existence only eighty yards from the end, the discovery of cooking would be, at most, fourteen feet from the end, and the development of agriculture would occur about four inches before our time. Coca-Cola would appear roughly 1/200th of an inch in the past!

For nearly the whole length of this road, our predecessors ate only whatever they could find or catch, and ate it the way they found it. Food processing wasn't invented yet. They also necessarily chose their food the way any animal except man still does today: by smell and taste. If its smell and taste were attractive, they moved toward it; and if they were unattractive, they moved away. Human babies respond this way, as do chimpanzees in the wild, our nearest genetic cousins. Neither possesses nutritional theories or taboos, nor modifies their food before it goes in their mouths. Their responses are instinctive; they are the fruits of evolution.

The human brain is organized on different levels corresponding to different periods of life evolution. Some of its most ancient structures are the hypothalamus and limbic system, also known as the primitive or reptilian brain because of our phylogenetic heritage from distant reptilian ancestors. These structures are common to all vertebrates, and organize basic survival behaviors and their related functions. They are automatic, built-in, and to a large extent operate independently of learning from experience. They are what we commonly call "instincts." For all species, they have always been the guarantee of well being and top fitness.

Over millions of years, the process of natural selection ensured the survival only of those species that were adapted to their environments. In biochemical terms, the survivors were those whose genetic codes (DNA) had programmed their individual organisms to detect, select, ingest, digest, and metabolize the kinds of available foods they needed to survive and to instinctively avoid natural poisons.

It is thanks to their built-in, DNA-programmed sensory systems that bees are attracted to flowers, cows to grass and squirrels to nuts, enabling these creatures to get exactly the foods their bodies are adapted to. The scheme of the universe, whatever it may be, was in play long before the emergence of the human neo-cortical capacity to analyze it . . . or to tamper with it.

Is humankind genetically adapted to Coke, French fries or other processed foods? These questions should not be taken lightly. The time spans involved in evolutionary processes are enormous. Since the advent of cooking, but particularly since the development of agriculture, humans have been altering their foods in increasingly complex ways. Have we, as a species, had time to genetically adapt to recently-introduced food products? Have our genes mutated so that we can safely handle the novel molecules contained in those "new" food products? The increasing number of studies that demonstrate a clear link between nutrition and disease indicate they haven't. While it is certainly true that "man does not live by bread alone," the real question is, can he live by bread at all? Upsetting as it may be, the answer seems to be, "No."

Genefit Nutrition is also based on the discovery that when a human being eats any food in its strictly original state, its taste changes at some point from pleasant to unpleasant. When the body's need for that particular food has been fulfilled, it no longer wants any more, even though it may still be hungry for other foods. However, this mechanism functions only with foods that have not been denatured in any way, and only when eaten separately, i.e., unmixed with others. This phenomenon does not occur with foods that have been frozen, cooked, chopped, or ground, or with extracts such as juices or oils. In nature, what an animal wants is one and the same as what it needs. Consequently, when dealing with foods whose structures evolved concurrently over millions of years with our own, our genetically determined senses of smell and taste tell us not only what we need, but also how much. And indeed, according to decades of experimentation, they do so very accurately. Obviously, the taste of a food is not to be found in the food itself, but in the perception of whoever is eating it. What a person needs, and therefore what he perceives as attractive, depends on the overall molecular state of his body at that particular moment. For example, we seek water only when we're thirsty, and instinctively stop drinking when we've had enough. Could we not expect this ability to apply to food as well? With strictly unprocessed food, it does. This is demonstrably true, and in a moment we will show you how you can prove it for yourself.

Once food is processed in any way, it goes beyond the capacity of our "instinctive computer" to analyze it. This is because cooking or otherwise modifying a food alters its original molecular structure, to which we are genetically adapted. Once cooked, it will taste the same indefinitely because its thermally modified structure will no longer trigger a taste-change response. The taste no longer changes because our sensory system has developed over millions of years in contact with the chemistry of strictly unprocessed food. Our instinctive brain centers are unable to correctly decode this altered chemical information brought in the form of recently introduced or denatured food. The reality is, we rarely if ever eat foods that can be evaluated instinctively. As a consequence, we can continue to eat it with whatever satisfaction it provides until we're full, and ingest many times the amount we actually required, which can lead to obesity and a host of other common afflictions.

Because human digestive enzymes originally adapted to the molecular structures of our native alimentary spectrum, which consisted of exclusively and strictly unprocessed foods, they cannot correctly process the novel molecular structures produced by culinary arts. Cooking, or any other type of processing, produces new chemical substances, also called NCC (new chemical compound), which did not exist until humans began to transform food. Anyone who doubts that cooking alters the molecular structure of food need only observe an egg white in the frying pan as it becomes opaque.

Our bodies should perhaps, at least in theory, be able to eliminate unnatural substances we are not adapted to and which may therefore be toxic to us. Unfortunately, observation repetitively showed us that we end up with toxic surpluses and accumulations of abnormal molecules in our tissues and even inside our cells. In a sense, we "make do" with modified foods, which we cannot metabolize properly.

During the course of detoxification periods triggered by Genefit

Nutrition, you may experience specific body odors reminding you of the cheese, mustard, or cooked foods eaten years before. But, after a time on Genefit Nutrition, once most abnormal molecules have been eliminated, feces, urine, and sweat drastically loose their unpleasant odor. The absence of abnormal odors can also be observed in animals living in the wild, which feed exclusively on unprocessed food. Hunters know by experience that deer feces or those of many other wild animals have hardly any odor.

Furthermore, it has been observed again and again that when a person is applying the principles of Genefit Nutrition for a longer period of time, and experiences, for instance, a viral infection, waste materials ejected by the body once more carry the odor of past meals of processed foods. These observations rather suggest that what is considered an illness at first may instead be a cleansing process. Consequently, it makes sense to think of certain microbes and viruses, not as "dangerous" pathogenic agents, but as having a very different function; if they are present during the time of detoxification, their presence could be misinterpreted as the cause of the problem instead of the results of the accumulation of unnatural molecules in the body. This view of pathogenic agents is a departure from current medical philosophy, which is based on observations of sickness and health exclusively in persons who have been exposed from birth to abnormal molecules, the end-products of denatured nutrients, with no understanding of their effects or even of their existence. Current medical thinking reflects a metaphysics of the enemy without versus the defenders within. But life is not that simple.

The human body is made up of some sixty trillion cells. They are of different types and sizes, but if we imagine a cell the size of a two-story house, a protein molecule would be comparable to a beer can, and an atom the size of a dust mote. Glucose passing through the intestinal mucous membrane does so at the rate of 100,000 billion molecules per second per square centimeter. The number of electro-chemical processes occurring in an organism at any moment is beyond our comprehension, so we must simplify our understanding of them to suit the capacities of our intellects. We take note of some things and neglect others, and postulate theories on the basis of what we've noticed and considered important. There's no crime here unless we forget that nature contains more than we can ever see or imagine. Our life processes, however we may represent them, are infinitely more complex than our "intelligence" (and its representations) to which they give rise, hence the need for greater respect for nature than we usually show.

From a Genefit Nutrition viewpoint, common diseases fall into two general categories:

1. those whose symptoms follow a very precise, predictable, and uniform pattern, such as measles, diphtheria, smallpox, and typhoid;
2. those that follow no coherent sequence — the ones that strike randomly, including cardiovascular diseases, cancers, multiple sclerosis, and psoriasis.

Under strict Genefit eating conditions, the symptoms of the first category of diseases are so benign as to be practically undetectable. You will discover this yourself if you consistently eat this way. When nutrition consists of genetically appropriate foods, a bout of flu will usually show very minor symptoms, and at the same time, often will be associated with the odor-charged (usually "rotten" or cheese-like) material extruded in sweat, urine, and feces that reveals its cleansing nature. This is true of most "diseases" whose symptoms follow predictable patterns and include odiferous discharges. Symptoms of such diseases are often more severe in people on traditional processed food diets because of the accumulations of abnormal molecules in the body's cells, tissues, and organs. The symptoms are further amplified by denatured food ingested during the course of the illness. In general, symptoms are proportional to the degree of past and present intoxication. In many cases medicine has no other choice than to put an end to the supposedly pathological processes, by suppressing or suspending the detoxification process. But such therapies preclude the system clean-out that would constitute a true cure. We will discuss these "patterned illnesses" in greater depth in later chapters, and we will show how many of these chronic or acute conditions can be healed simply by eliminating processed foods from the diet. As we will see, true and long-lasting health can only be achieved when the body is clear of abnormal and unnatural molecules.

The second class of diseases in this frame of reference is the class of diseases that have no set pattern. They are also, to a great extent, a consequence of toxic accumulations the body was unable to eliminate. It is generally known and readily admitted, for instance, that a number of insecticides, food preservatives and coloring agents, and synthetic sweeteners may produce cancers and/or other severe pathological conditions in laboratory animals, and should therefore not be used by humans. It has also been shown that many of these substances, antibiotics among them, accumulate in animal and human tissues. It is apparent, however, that any substance which is too alien to be either fully used or discarded by the body's biochemistry will accumulate and may have some degree of pathological effect. New chemical substances produced by food processing are no exception, since the human body hasn't had time to genetically and biochemically adapt to them. Will the pathology or the potential for pathology disappear once the new chemical substances are removed both from the body and from daily meals? That is essentially what happens when Genefit Nutrition is applied correctly, unless the pathology has gone too far and organs have been irreversibly damaged.

If you decide to eat by instinct, you will probably be in for some pleasant surprises. Normally, if you do it correctly, within two or three days, any digestive problem you had will disappear. Within a few weeks, most chronic pain and discomforts will have subsided or disappeared completely, including stiff neck, inflammatory pain, arthritic pain, migraines, and so on. This claim may seem unbelievable, but, as you will see for yourself, it is so. Once they have eliminated the first part of denatured-food toxins from their bodies, instinctively nourished people even become immune to the inflammatory pain after a burn or a cut, except for the few minutes of physical pain immediately following the accident.

You can also expect nervous problems to subside dramatically after only a few days on Genefit Nutrition, although you may experience transient crises as abnormal molecules are being eliminated from your body tissues via your bloodstream or lymphatic system. But in a short time most nervousness and irritability will have gone, and you will experience an improved psycho-physiological state as well as an increased ability to face problems with equanimity. This calming effect is particularly noticeable in animals, who have no expectations or preconceived notions. As we will see later in this book, when animals are switched from a processed food environment to an unprocessed one or vice versa, their overall behavior is considerably modified. Unfortunately, the effect of neuroactive and neurotoxic molecules contained in processed foods is still greatly underestimated.

With Genefit Nutrition you will become much healthier than the average "healthy" person. You can expect to feel more energetic with less sleep. You can expect to lose your excess fat at a rate of up to one pound a day and you will then stabilize at your ideal weight after some time. If you apply the principles of Genefit Nutrition correctly, you will not be as susceptible to colds and flu symptoms or subject to hypoglycemic mood swings. Eating by instinct will prevent infections in wounds whose healing time will be about half what is "normal."

Women who have been consistently eating the Genefit way can expect to experience symptom-free periods, a stabilization of their cycle, and no transitioning difficulties during menopause. A majority of women applying Genefit Nutritional principles precisely over longer periods of time report little or no pain when giving birth, and the pushing state of labor is likely to be a matter of minutes rather than hours. Furthermore, the waters break at the end of the process rather than at the beginning, so that the baby is propelled hydraulically through the birth canal. This phenomenon has been observed many times, and is presumably what nature intended, as opposed to what unnatural nutrition prevents.

Genefit Nutrition has been applied successfully in cases of severe pathologies including cataracts, herpes, colitis, psoriasis, asthma, allergies, diabetes, staphylococcal infections, and ulcers. It has saved the lives of cancer and leukemia patients, ended tremor and paralysis in persons with multiple sclerosis, and eliminated pain in patients with arthritis and glaucoma.

And still it is very important to note that Genefit Nutrition *does not cure*. The exclusion of food processing offers an opportunity to rid the body of all the possible disturbance factors at once and allow it to function the way it did during most of our evolutionary history. Because genetically inappropriate food can make us sick, its total absence from our daily diet produces numerous improvements and recoveries. A number of case histories and reports are included in later chapters, providing examples of what genetically proper nutrition can do.

Within your own body, you will experience simple cause-and-effect relationships between food and health, which will create a sense of self-empowerment. Rather than depending on ever-changing approaches to health and well being you will find the answers within yourself and be able to actively influence the state of your body and mind.

In addition to its success when applied to diverse pathologies, adopting Genefit Nutrition is a life-changing experience. It will literally change the way you perceive the world and the way you relate to it in a powerful, positive way.

By now you might be saying to yourself: it sounds too good to be true. And, if it is true, why didn't anybody discover it before? One answer to this question is: tradition. No culture exists on earth at this time — nor has any existed for many thousands of years — that does not mix, season, cook, or otherwise denature its foods. Food processing has become a planetary phenomenon, and cooking, in particular, is everywhere assumed to be not only natural, but necessary. Research in medicine and nutrition has rarely, if ever, questioned this premise. So the concept that abnormal molecules, to which we are not genetically adapted, accumulate in the body, and the fact that we possess a nutritional instinct which only functions normally with foods in their original, unmodified state, was necessarily a long time in coming.

NOTES

1. S. Jones, R. Martin, D.Pilbeam, "The Cambridge Encyclopedia of Human Evolution," Cambridge University Press 1999, 2.7 p.72.

2. Zhao Z, Jin L, Fu YX, Ramsay M, Jenkins T, Leskinen E, Pamilo P, Trexler M, Patthy L, Jorde LB, Ramos-Onsins S, Yu N, Li WH, "Worldwide DNA sequence variation in a 10-kilobase noncoding region on human chromosome 22." Proc Natl Acad Sci U S A 2000 Oct 10;97(21):11354-8.

3. Deaths and death rates for the 10 leading causes of death in specified age groups, by race and sex: United States, 1998, *National Vital Statistics Reports*, Vol. 48, No. 11, July 24, 2000.

TWO

A Question of Adaptation

"Science is common sense at its best."

— *Aldous Huxley*

TO WHAT KIND OF FOOD are we genetically adapted? This is, in fact, a very simple, but nevertheless fundamental question. An engine is built to use a specific type of fuel (diesel, gasoline, kerosene, etc.). To ensure optimal performance and longevity, we need to use the fuel the engine was built for. But, how can a car owner be sure he puts the right type of fuel in his car? The easiest way to find out is to consult the manufacturer's user manual, which gives us all the technical specifications of the engine. If we apply the same method to living matter, from all we know today, we can surely consider DNA to be the "manufacturer's user manual" of our biological engine.

DNA is our cellular "information system," containing the instructions for our reproductive, digestive, and metabolic processes and for practically everything else that goes on in our bodies. The amount of information it contains is enormous. Figuratively speaking, the DNA in a single cell holds as much electrochemically coded data as all the books in an entire public library. It is encoded in the form of a double helix, whose sequential molecular arrangement is peculiar to each species. If the length of DNA from one cell were to be uncoiled and stretched out straight, it would be nearly six feet long. With our trillions of cells, we each contain enough DNA to stretch around the world five million times. DNA, the code of life that will provide us with the most accurate answers to our fundamental question.

The information contained in DNA is just beginning to be decoded. The process is painstaking. Yet we can already conclude that, in general, characteristics that are common to a class of organisms are most commonly determined by their DNA. In this regard, everyone agrees that a lion eats meat and a cow eats mainly grass and not vice versa. A lion would not survive eating grass exclusively. Every species has its dietary spectrum prescribed by its genetic makeup. No animal consciously chooses the food it is meant to eat. It is simply attracted to one food rather than another, mostly by its sense of smell. The key to this attraction lies in its DNA, and consequently, is preset prior to birth. The lion, for example, is genetically adapted to digest and live on meat. A lion doesn't get sick when it regularly eats meat for which it has adapted over millions of years; otherwise, the species would have become extinct long ago or undergone adaptive mutations. As a matter of fact, the genetic mutation of any species both produces and results from changes in the overall structure of the biological plenum. Various models exist to explain how mutations may occur and become self-perpetuating. All point to the conclusion that "life" is an ongoing experiment, and that any species that does not mutate in such a way as to adapt to its changing environment will perish. Lions obviously survived, and after having been submitted to harsh evolutionary pressures, lions became genetically adapted to meat at three different levels:

1. A metabolic level, in the sense that it possess the appropriate intestines and enzymes needed to digest meat — all the complex cellular biology needed to assimilate and use nutrients and proteins contained in meat in a safe and efficient manner.
2. A biological level, in the sense that it has all the "weapons" necessary to kill and catch its prey. Long teeth and claws are evidently also the product of the lion's genetic adaptation to its environment.
3. An instinctual level, in the sense that it has all the instincts to hunt and has a food-intake regulation mechanism assuring optimum dietary balance needed to survive in the wild.

As one can see with the example of the lion, the question of genetic adaptation to food is relatively easy to answer when we are talking about animals; all we have to do is observe them in their natural habitat for some time, and then we can draw conclusions about their diet in relation to their genetic makeup.

But now, what about us?

Approaching the problem of finding humans' most healthy diet through genetics and evolution gives a whole new perspective, which happens to strongly challenge traditional ways of thinking about nutrition and dietetics. In fact, there can be no accurate science of nutrition without the question of genetic adaptation taken into consideration. This question should be the very base of dietetics. Unfortunately, it isn't. Although the idea of a possible mismatch between modern processed foods and our genes may not be accepted by most professionals in medicine and dietetics, it has nonetheless been around for almost thirty years, especially in the small scientific circles of nutritional anthropology. Even if there is a slowly growing interest in this approach, questioning a fundamental assumption of civilization isn't easy, and such a revolutionary concept does not win acceptance overnight. At the same time, how can we claim to set the standards of nutrition if we do not consider the historical conditions in which our bodies have evolved?

It is sometimes argued that humans must have become adapted to denatured foods, because if we weren't, as a species, we wouldn't have survived to this day. True? Not true? The question definitely warrants exploration. There is no doubt that we make do with processed foods, but at a price, as we will see later in this book. However, are we genetically adapted to them?

As far as the pace of genetic adaptation over time is concerned, first there is a concept that needs to be clarified. We speak imprecisely when we say a species has adapted or not adapted to certain conditions. Adaptation is a matter of degree. Even respected researchers use the term "adapted" in this inexact way, as though we were always either completely adapted or not adapted at all. Here, we cannot think in terms of yes or no. Genetic adaptation to a specific food can be unachieved or partial. We can be adapted to some molecules in that given food, while other molecules contained in the same food can remain harmful. Similarly, we may be partially adapted to some molecules, in the sense that they are disadvantageous at this stage in our evolution, but not extremely so. A more complete adaptation may take many generations. In the meantime, this specific food may still present a health risk.

With food processing, such as cooking and the recent introduction of dairy products and cereals, we aren't facing just a single toxic molecule, which already takes an enormous amount of time for a species to adapt, but, as we will see later in this chapter, we are confronted with a huge array of new chemical substances that have entered the dietary spectrum within a very short period of time. We must have adapted to some of them to some degree and to others to a lesser degree. To be able to conclude that we are genetically adapted to our current traditional diet, it is very important for this adaptation to be achieved. Otherwise, all we do is adjust and make do with a food environment that does not match our physiology.

For example, with the advent of agriculture and animal husbandry, Northern Europeans have consumed cow's milk products into adulthood for the past ten thousand years. As a result, the digestive system of Northern Europeans is able to provide a lifelong production of lactase, an enzyme necessary to digest lactose, which is a carbohydrate contained in cow's milk. In Asians and Africans the production of lactase ceases by the age of four or five. This condition is not surprising, since the body naturally produces lactase for the sole purpose of digesting mother's milk. Because cow's milk products are not traditionally a part of the Asian's and most Africans' diet, they have consequently not adapted to them; they are unable to digest cow's milk properly and quickly suffer from many symptoms after its consumption. As soon as the discovery of a lifelong production of lactase was made, some people erroneously concluded that Northern Europeans must have genetically adapted to cow's milk. Yet, more and more scientific studies revealing health problems generated by cow's milk indicate that the adaptation of Northern Europeans to cow's milk is incomplete enough to still be unsafe. In fact, Northern Europeans only evolved enough so that adults can handle lactose, which is only one of the many chemical elements in cow's milk. Since lactose is a carbohydrate also present in mother's milk, it was a small adaptive step for the body to prolong the production of lactase. Casein, on the other hand, a protein also found in cow's milk, generates immunologic intolerance in almost every newborn baby, which strongly suggests that humans are not genetically equipped to handle casein, a substance that doesn't appear in mother's milk. Casein is a completely foreign protein, the digestion of which would require deep changes at an enzymatic and genomic level. A few decades ago, instead of questioning the consumption of cow's milk itself for newborn babies, laboratories came up with hypoallergenic formula, presumably making cow's milk more "tolerable."

Whether to take another species' milk, alter food, or make the simplest recipes, the use of conceptual intelligence is indispensable. In order to invent recipes, one needs to conceptualize action in the future, and to remember past intentions. These are the same capacities needed for making tools. Tool-making goes back approximately two million years, with *homo abilitis* showing the first true signs of conceptual intelligence. No recipe could have been invented prior to the creation of tools, even the uncooked ones. For all animals, the conceptualization of a recipe is still impossible. Human intelligence, on the other hand, made it possible for us to become the only species on the planet that artificially processes food, in many complex ways. The resulting dietary spectrum of modern humans is not a natural one.

Cooking, for instance, is an exclusively human artifact. Despite much research, there is still controversy about exactly when humankind started cooking. Hearths have been found on sites occupied by *hominids* about four hundred thousand years ago, but those sites do not tell much about cooking itself. It is probable that fire was used for protection from predators at first. If there was cooking involved, was it occasional, seasonal, or regular? We don't know. Such sites are exceptional. Hearths are not common in the archaeological records until about forty thousand years ago, when the ability to make fire had surely been acquired on a widespread basis.[1] It has been hypothesized that cooking goes back 1.9 million years. Those theories are speculative and have not been supported by any subsequent archeological records. The fact is, we don't know for sure when our ancestors began cooking food on a regular basis—a basis that would have caused enough evolutionary pressure for the body to adapt. We can only estimate. What we do know is that with the beginning of agriculture around ten thousand years ago at the period commonly called the Neolithic, our ancestors underwent drastic changes in dietary habits within a very short period of time. The beginning of agriculture and animal husbandry with the use of grinding equipment, pots, ovens, and the consumption of dairy products, grains, and cereals also marks the beginning of culinary art.

When looking back at our evolutionary history, we might mistakenly assume that evolutionary adaptation is quite a simple and straightforward process, unless we realize the time spans involved. Our evolutionary road is so long that it is virtually beyond our understanding. Humankind's oldest recorded history goes back only a few thousand years, and the archeological remains of "ancient" civilizations are hardly any older. For most of us, however, the "dawn of civilization" happened too long ago to even try to think back to. The two hundred-odd years that have elapsed since the creation of the United States already seem like a "very long time" to most of us. So, we have trouble grasping the fact that men and women very much like ourselves were already walking the earth not only two thousand or twenty thousand years ago, but two hundred thousand and even two million years ago. Already, six million years ago, our ancestors came down from the trees and very gradually, one generation after another they finally became us.

At most, ten thousand years, representing only 0.16 percent of our six million-year-old evolutionary history, have elapsed since our ancestors first began to plant seeds and keep domestic animals. On the other hand, geneticists know that a species-wide genetic adaptation to a new food environment happens very slowly. Widespread significant genetic changes can be found only within a time frame of a million to several million years.

Recent comparative studies between paleontology and genetics have shown that adaptation time is extremely long. One can compare genes of related living species whose date of origin is comparatively well known. What one notices is that the number of mutations that separate the corresponding genes is approximately proportional to the time elapsed between the dates when the species first appeared (at which time mutations occurred).

In the graph below, the horizontal axis records the date of origin of the species under review. On the vertical axis, the number of mutations that distinguish the different species are provided. In this way, sloping lines indicate the rate of mutation per time unit (G. Hervé, *The Evolution of Proteins* [Masson, 1983], 16).

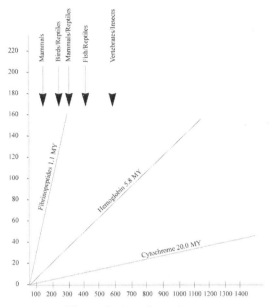

FIGURE 1. The evolution of proteins.

The times necessary for mutations changing
1 percent of genes are the following:

1) The gene encoded for fibrinopeptides (proteins involved
   in coagulation): 1.1 million years
2) The gene encoded for hemoglobin: 5.8 million years
3) The gene encoded for cytochrome C: 20 million years
4) The gene encoded for histones IV: 1000 million years

Paleontological remains indicate the first use of fire at no more than four
hundred thousand years ago. But in terms of evolutionary time-spans,
four hundred thousand years ago is "yesterday," and ten thousand years is
"a moment ago." It seems that *Homo sapiens'* parental apes could not
have been adapted to milk, bread, or roast beef, simply because, over the
seventy million years of their evolutionary development, such foods as
these were never part of their diet.

Today, thanks to the science of chemistry, we know that any type of
food processing creates chemical reactions that change the chemical for-

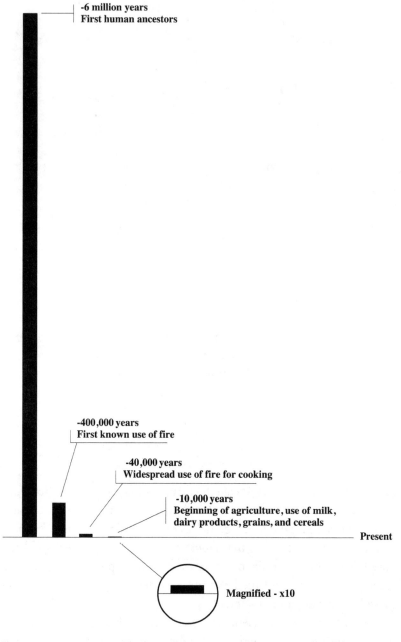

FIGURE 2. Time comparison between human evolution and major changes in dietary habits.

mula and structure of a given food. At some point in our past, the chemical composition of food changed drastically, because of the introduction of processing techniques and new varieties of foods. If we compare the time frame within which those dietary changes occurred to the time needed to adapt to them, it is completely legitimate to state the hypothesis that food processing is much too recent for a genetic adaptation to have been achieved.

Because of the molecular agitation generated by heat, cooking produces millions of unpredictable carbohydrate/protein combinations, commonly called Maillard molecules. A kitchen is nothing more than a chemical laboratory producing millions of novel chemical substances that are not present in the natural world, or at best may appear very rarely, by accident. During most of our evolutionary history, before food processing, human beings never ingested close to the amount of Maillard molecules that we ingest nowadays. In addition, it was only ten thousand years ago that dairy products and cereals were introduced into the dietary spectrum of humans, also bringing new foreign molecules, which weren't there before. And finally, only one hundred years ago, at the beginning of the industrial age, the food industry gave birth to even more foreign chemicals in the form of additives, preservatives, food moisturizers, etc. Throughout human culinary history, most of these new chemicals were introduced without anyone seriously worrying about whether they matched our bodies' genetic characteristics, and therefore, our physiology's ability to handle them safely. Nevertheless, in recent years, the harmfulness of some of these chemical substances has begun to be pointed out. Chemists and researchers have identified some of those new molecules as being:

1. Toxic; that is, they act as poisons in the body.

    In 1975, Adrian and Susbielle showed that heating glycol (an elemental amino acid) with glucose released pre-melanoidins (Maillard molecules), which are toxic for a rat embryo.
    All it took was blending the compound with the food ration of pregnant rats, in a one-to-six ratio, for the average number of births per litter to drop by 45 percent. Other researchers like Chelius et al., Stegink, and Pitkin also noted the presence of pre-melanoidins in fetal blood when the mother was fed a supplement of it. Lederer and Dushimimana, the co-authors of this

article, heated a mixture of glucose (the most widespread sugar) and lysine (one of the eight basic amino acids) for two hours at a temperature of 90°C, by which time, 50 percent of both compounds had reacted, forming random, abnormal molecules (Maillards molecules). When they blended the compound with the feed of pregnant rats in a one-to-six ratio, the following results were obtained:

1) The number of embryos per litter was down from 9.80 to 3.75.

2) Embryonic weight and placental weight decreased and increased respectively. The researchers read the results as poisoning rather than dietary deficiency. In the same vein, Kuhler et al. have shown that dietary deficiency induces both weight loss in embryos and weight gain in placentas.

3) Moreover, the researchers reported teratogenic vascularized tumor of the navel. This is a most serious malformation so far only attested in rats that had been administered trypan blue coloring (Gillman et al.), or who were severely deficient in folic acid (Nelson et al.), or who were massively dosed with streptonigrine salicylates (Warkany and Takacs) (J. Lederer and A. Dushimimana, "Molecules heated in cooking generate compounds toxic for embryos," *Cahiers de nutrition et de dietetique (Journal of nutrition and diet)*, March 1982: 36-37).

2. Carcinogenic; that is, they are involved in the production of cancer cells.

Carcinogens occur naturally in the foods we eat, including a number of HCAs that have been identified in foods (beef, pork, poultry and fish) as a result of cooking. These compounds are formed during the normal cooking process by the reaction of creatine with various amino acids. The HCAs have been identified as a result of their high mutagenic activity in the Ames test. The HCAs can be separated into two types, the nonimidazole and the imidazole type, the latter of which is the predominant type present in Western foods. Both types of HCAs have been found to be carcinogenic in rodent bioassays. Of the three imidazole compounds presently under evaluation in nonhuman primates, one has been found to be a potent carcinogen, inducing hepatocellular carcinoma in a majority of the animals in approximately one-seventh of their life span. In addition, a high proportion of the nonhuman primates also had focal IQ-induced myocardial lesions as observed by both light and electron microscopic findings. This information, along with other toxicology data on the HCAs, much of which is cited in this paper, allows the inference to be made that heterocyclic amines may be a risk factor for both cancer and cardiovascular disease in humans (R.H. Adamson and U.P. Thorgeirsson, *Carcinogens in foods: heterocyclic amines and Cancer and Heart disease*, Adv Exp Med Biol 1995;369:211-20).

3. Mutagenic; that is, they disturb the DNA replication process and produce unpredictable mutations.

Mutation assay with Salmonella typhimurium enabled us to detect various types of mutagens in cooked foods. A series of mutagenic heterocyclic amines has been isolated and identified in broiled fish and meat and in pyrolyzates of amino acids and proteins. Feeding experiments showed these mutagens to be carcinogenic in mice and rats. The mechanism of formation and pathway of metabolic activation of these heterocyclic amines have been elucidated. Their contents in various cooked foods have been determined. The presence of mutagenic nitropyrenes (some of which were confirmed as carcinogens) in grilled chicken was also established. Roasted coffee beans also yield mutagens such as methylglyoxal. The formation of mutagen precursors, including beta-carboline derivatives and tyramine which become mutagens with nitrite treatment, was found during food processing. Oncogene activation in animal tumors induced by some of these food mutagens/carcinogens has been confirmed. The role of mutagens/carcinogens in cooked foods in human cancer development has not yet been exactly evaluated. In order to do this, more information on their carcinogenic potency, human intake, metabolism in the human body, and the effects of combined administration with other initiators, promoters, and other modifying factors in food is required (T. Sugimura, "Past, present, and future of mutagens in cooked foods," *Environ. Health Perspectives* 1986 Aug; 67:5-10).

4. Neurotoxic; that is, they cause disturbances in the nerve centers of the brain.

During aging long-lived proteins accumulate specific post-translational modifications. One family of modifications, termed Maillard reaction products, are initiated by the condensation between amino groups of proteins and reducing sugars. Protein modification by the Maillard reaction is associated with crosslink formation, decreased protein solubility, and increased protease resistance. Here, we present evidence that the characteristic pathological structures associated with Alzheimer disease contain modifications typical of advanced Maillard reaction end products. Specifically, antibodies against two Maillard end products, pyrraline and pentosidine, immunocytochemically label neurofibrillary tangles and senile plaques in brain tissue from patients with Alzheimer disease. In contrast, little or no staining is observed in apparently healthy neurons of the same brain. The Maillard-reaction-related modifications described herein could account for the biochemical and insolubility properties of the lesions of Alzheimer disease through the formation of protein crosslinks (M.A. Smith, S.Taneda, P.L. Richey, S. Miyata, S.D. Yan , D. Stern, L.M. Sayre, V.M. Monnier, G. Perry,

"Advanced Maillard reaction end products are associated with Alzheimer disease pathology." *Proc Natl Acad Sci USA* 1994 Jun 7; 91(12):5710-4).

5. Antigenic; that is, they play a role in autoimmune diseases.

Rheumatoid arthritis (RA) is the commonest form of chronic inflammatory rheumatism. In France, it affects over 1 percent of individuals and around three women for every man. In spite of very great strides made in basic immunology, the mechanism for autoimmune diseases has not yet been brought to light. We believe that minute amounts of peptides, and even proteins, can make their way through the intestinal barrier. This phenomenon increases in certain circumstances: when intestinal mucus changes, when huge amounts of protein are eaten, and there's an enzymatic deficit of enterocytes.

The theory of enzymatic unsuitability to a new protein fits in well with the background surrounding RA. A modification, through one or more mutations, of a commonly eaten protein could explain the rather recent appearance of the disease.

As for the spread of RA in the nineteenth century, it could be accounted for by the worldwide distribution of food containing proteins that appeared recently through mutation.

In this study, we had patients who were clear cases of RA, according to ARA standards, go on a diet from which was excluded two non-initial substances eaten and drunk in huge amounts, wheat and milk, as well as all their byproducts.

We were able to bring together the results of the diet for twenty-four people who tried a diet exclusively consisting of unprocessed foods and using the nutritional instinct for at least three months. It must be pointed out that traditional therapy was not given up when patients took up the diet. Out of the 24 RA examined with the distance of at least three months, there were:

- 5 constant conditions
- 1 slight improvement
- 6 clear-up improvements
- 6 major improvements
- 6 full recoveries

Therefore, it seems advisable to search out the possible presence of suspicious peptides in various kinds of wheat protein and cow's milk. The positive effects of the diet not only involves morbid joint symptoms but, also, and quite significantly, the general and psychological condition of the patient. This preliminary study does not enable us to conclude that the first of those effects is not merely the consequence of the other two and, therefore, to conclude that the theory is valid. But the results are interesting enough to hope that research into that field will proceed ("Trying a diet without cereal grains and milk in cases of rheumatoid polyarthritis." Thesis submitted at the school of medicine in Montpellier by Helen Rouxin to qualify as a (medical) doctor in June 1989, excerpts).

Current research has uncovered more and more evidence that food processing, cooking, and the use of dairy products, grains, and cereals, present a serious threat to human health on a large scale. Every specialist working in a field somewhat related to nutrition knows that a molecule is considered toxic or harmful to the human body, if the body doesn't have the digestive enzymes to break it down properly, or, in other words, when the body is not genetically adapted to this particular type of molecule.

The hypothesis of a potential nonadaptation to modern processed foods needs to be taken seriously; knowing the huge difference between the time period in which drastic dietary changes occurred and the actual time needed to adapt to them, how can we be sure that degenerative diseases and other major and minor health problems in modern civilization do not come from a possible nonadaptation? Every time we are confronted with a health problem, we would do well to ask ourselves whether it is part of the natural human condition and to be accepted as is, or the result of a mismatch between what we eat and our body's genetic makeup.

So far, the science of genetics has been unable to tell us if we are safely adapted to processed foods or not for a very simple reason: in order for geneticists to determine how long it might take for us to adapt to changes in our diet, they would need to know to what precisely we should have adapted to. Since food chemists and toxicologists have been unable to index and classify the astronomical number of different molecules produced by cooking alone, how could any one come up with an accurate time frame required for an adequate adaptation? Amazing as it sounds, despite all our research and technology, we still don't know what is really going on in a cooking pot!

There are cases, however, in which the connection between food processing and sickness is clear. Thanks to epidemiological research, the consensus among health professionals is that heated fats are involved in the development of cardiovascular diseases. But, what about other foods? According to the Cancer Epidemiology Services at the New Jersey Department of Health and Senior Services, in 1996, out of a U.S. population sample of 100,000 people, there were 40,085 reported cases of cancer. With two persons out of five in the U. S. subject to cancer, the question of genetic adaptation is vitally important.

> "Maps of cancer are potentially very informative because they provide one kind of evidence of how much cancer is, in principle, avoidable," says Michael Thun, M.D., vice president for epidemiology and surveillance research for the American Cancer Society (ACS).
>
> Those variations were first analyzed in detail in 1981, when an Oxford University report commissioned by the U.S. Congress came out. It tracked cancer worldwide and found 70 percent to 80 percent is caused by environmental factors. That doesn't mean only environmental pollution, however. Epidemiologists use the term "environmental" to describe all the factors other than the genes one is born with, Thun says.
>
> The Oxford study looked at differences among different countries, and within countries. For example, stomach cancer, now rare in the U.S., is extremely common in certain parts of China. However, researchers believe that differences in food types, methods of food preservation, and chronic infection with Helicobacter pylori account for most of the variation in stomach cancer incidence rates ("Web Site Maps U.S. Cancer Deaths by Region" American Cancer Society; Article date: 2001/03/09).

We can consider ourselves adapted to a food only under specific conditions: this food should not present any health hazard when consumed on a regular basis, over a long period of time, by a significant number of people. As we mentioned, lions don't get sick from eating meat for which they have adapted over millions of years; neither do cows while eating grass for which they have adapted in the same manner. Many studies have demonstrated that humans' health, on the other hand, can be negatively affected by the regular consumption of French fries, cooked meat, and other processed foods. As long as we have proof that a given food presents any threat for health, or even produces the slightest recurrent symptoms, it seems clear that our body doesn't know how to handle it chemically. Therefore, we can conclude that we are not genetically adapted to it. In more general terms, as long as some individuals contract food-related diseases, we, as a species, cannot consider ourselves completely adapted to our current diet. Numerous pathologies from cancer to Alzheimer's disease have proven to be food-related, and more specifically, *cooking*-related. There are many other diseases that should be studied from this perspective, otherwise medical practitioners will never have a clear picture about their etiology.

This discussion leads us to the conclusion that we are currently in the process of adaptation to cooked foods. It seems that the human species is currently subject to a process of natural selection through the elimination of individuals who do not handle the novel food environment well. Natural selection eliminates individuals of a given species before they are able to pass their DNA to the next generation; this is how adaptation takes place. There is approximately 0.1 percent genetic variability among our species[2]; some individuals' genetic make-up probably suits processed food better than others. But, if we are still in the process of adaptation, approximately seven hundred thousand deaths a year from cardiovascular diseases and approximately five hundred thousand deaths a year from cancer in the U.S. alone[3] might be the price we currently pay for that adaptation to happen. Is it worth it? The choice is ours.

In a distant future, the human species will probably achieve adaptation to processed food. There are nonetheless two issues that might dramatically slow the process down. The first is the occurrence of ever-changing recipes and processing techniques. New recipes and new processing techniques produce new classes of toxic molecules, to which the body needs time to adapt. For a genetic adaptation to be achieved in response to a changing dietary factor, that factor would have to be constant over generations. However, this is not the case with culinary art! For example, the introduction of new foods cooked in different manners at different temperatures for different lengths of time would necessarily produce different thermally generated compounds. So, a genetic adaptation to a wide selection of heat-modified foods is unlikely to occur. The second issue is, ironically . . . modern medicine. Medicine saves the lives of those who are less adapted and in doing so, it allows the less adapted DNA to make it to the next generation where similar health problems will again be confronted. Considering the amplitude of this phenomenon, more research is needed. The better we understand the process of adaptation or nonadaptation with regard to food processing, the greater will be our ability to prevent health problems.

If we now conclude that we might not be adapted to everything we eat, we need to ask ourselves: What foods are more likely to match our body's genetic make-up? Fortunately, there are some facts that point towards an answer:

Humans and apes are in many ways very similar. The structure of the digestive tracts of humans and chimpanzees is almost identical. We carry the same sorts of intestinal flora, and we harbor many of the same diseases and viruses. Amazingly, our genetic codes are almost identical. Various approaches have been used for determining the "genetic distance" between species. Comparisons have been made between humans and apes using behavioral, anatomical, physiological, and other criteria. On a molecular level, the determination involves a structural comparison of our DNA. More than ninety-eight percent of a human DNA string is identical to that of a chimpanzee. In fact, from a geneticist's point of view, we are closer to chimpanzees than chimpanzees are to gorillas.

> Some of the amino acid sequences in humans were virtually identical with those of apes such as the chimpanzee or gorilla . . .
>
> The sequences of human and chimpanzee polypeptides examined to date are, on the average, more than 99 percent identical (Mary-Claire King and A.C. Wilson, "Evolution at Two Levels in Humans and Chimpanzees." *Science*, Val. 188 No.4184, April 11, 1975).

Two six-foot lengths of human and chimpanzee DNA strings laid side-by-side fail to match one another over only a little bit more than one inch of their length. Our biological closeness to chimpanzees is such that when a veterinarian cares for a sick chimpanzee, he or she often consults a physician. The reverse also holds true; when researchers want to study the etiology of any particular disease, they often use chimpanzees as a model, because of this amazing closeness.

Among primatologists, it is well known that our cousins, the chimpanzees, are clearly not adapted to processed foods. Chimpanzees in captivity suffer pathologies similar to our own. When the first chimpanzees were brought to laboratories and zoos, many of them died of pneumonia, diabetes, and many other diseases after only a few years of captivity. To solve that problem, modern researchers and zookeepers tried feeding chimpanzees a diet that was as close as possible to what they eat in the wild: unprocessed fruits and greens. With this change, mortality rates in captivity have dropped sharply.

Humans and chimpanzees share exactly the same digestive enzymes. In fact, there have been no digestive enzymes found in humans that are not also present in chimpanzees. This finding not only strongly suggests that we humans have not adapted to processed food much more than chimpanzees have, but also that we are still adapted to a similar diet based exclusively on unprocessed foods.

It may not be totally correct to assume that the differentiation between humans and chimpanzees has been growing at a steady rate, because some "quantum jump" mutations may well have occurred along the way. But if we assume a steady evolutionary rate, then the gulf between us and chimpanzees has been widening at the rate of only 22/100ths of one percent per million years. So that in the 400,000 years, at most, since man began using fire for cooking, less than 1/10th of one percent of our DNA code would be expected to have evolved in response to the novel nutritional molecules so produced.

> The human genetic constitution has changed relatively little since the appearance of truly modern human beings, Homo sapiens sapiens, about 40,000 years ago. Even the development of agriculture 10,000 years ago has apparently had a minimal influence on our genes . . .
> Such developments as the Industrial Revolution, agribusiness, and modern food-processing techniques have occurred too recently to have had any evolutionary effect at all. Accordingly, the range of diets available to preagricultural human beings determines the range that still exists for men and women living in the 20th century - the nutrition for which human beings are in essence genetically programmed (S.B. Eaton and M. Konner, "Paleolithic Nutrition,"*The New England Journal of Medicine*, Jan., 1985).

From an evolutionary point of view, our physiological and digestive functions, like those of any other animal, adapted over millions of years to the chemistry of strictly unprocessed foods, provided directly by nature. In a time when food processing didn't exist, unprocessed foods were by default the only food available. When Lucy, one of the oldest skeletons of early humans ever found, took her first steps, there is no doubt about the fact that she fed on unprocessed, unaltered foods such as fruits, herbs, roots, and nuts, eating them one by one without mixing them, as chimpanzees still do today.

It is very important to keep in mind that the degree of adaptation to a specific food increases with the time of exposure. According to the archaeological record, as much as 99.34 percent of our evolution as human beings has occurred under an unprocessed food environment and only 0.66 percent represents the amount of time corresponding to the forty thousand-year period when cooking became widespread and common. Upon reviewing these numbers, there can be little doubt that a diet of strictly unprocessed foods is best suited to our genetic makeup. With this in mind, we can see that we have statistically far more chances to be adapted to an unprocessed food diet than to a traditional processed one. It is also interesting to consider that even if occasional food processing was the practice of our ancestors, they still remained on a diet partially, and sometimes mainly, composed of fruits, nuts, and vegetal products. In fact, we have never stopped eating them. They still are a part of our diet today.

> For better health, eat more like our pre-human ancestors, says an intriguing new study. Here's how.
>
> For two weeks, Tom Ransom ate like a prehistoric man. No potato chips or French fries. Just lots of fruits, vegetables and nuts. "I had to eat 20 pounds of fruits and vegetables a day," Ransom says, exaggerating the amount of fiber he ate, which was actually 100 grams a day. "I wouldn't say it was enjoyable, but tolerable."
>
> Although paleontologists do not know what our human-like ancestors who walked on two legs ate millions of years ago, the researchers say gathering available foodstuffs, such as greens and fruits, played a larger role in our early development than hunting small animals.
>
> DIET LOWERED CHOLESTEROL
>
> The study diet, which had a total of 2,500 calories, was high in fiber and did not have cholesterol-laden meats, cheese or butter implicated in heart disease. After one week on the diet, the researchers found those participants' bad cholesterol levels dropped by 33 percent. "The changes were very fast," says Dr. David Jenkins, a professor of nutritional science at St. Michael's Hospital of the University of Toronto and leader of the study. "We noticed significant changes within one week."

The decrease was more than with some cholesterol-lowering drugs, Jenkins says, and more than that of subjects eating the so-called Mediterranean diet of grains and starches, and the modern low-fat diet recommended by the American Heart Association.

The study results were published in the April 2001 issue of the medical journal Metabolism.

Fran Berkoff, a nutritionist with the Mount Sinai Hospital in Toronto, says the results underline the value of eating more soluble fiber, and fruits and vegetables (*What If We Ate Like Pre-humans?* Tuesday June 12 08:13 PM EDT 2001 *ABC News*).

In the course of traditional research, when a class of molecules contained in a food is suspected of being harmful to the human body, there are two main ways researchers may proceed. In the first protocol, they isolate the chemicals involved and then experiment on animals to observe the effects. The other protocol involves the utilization of epidemiological studies in which researchers test a sample of population with subjects who have been exposed to those molecules and compare symptoms with another population sample of subjects who have not been exposed to the chemicals. In both protocols, there is a premise — the assumption that a specific class of molecules or a specific food is toxic. But this assumption unavoidably limits the field of exploration; it can easily become the tree hiding the forest. Traditional nutritional studies compare the results of one group of processed foods with the results of another group of processed foods. An unhealthy diet including a certain food, when compared to an unhealthy diet of processed foods without that particular food, may demonstrate little or no difference in their results because important factors have been missed. The central hypothesis of Genefit Nutrition leads us to expect that processed foods in general contain chemicals to which we have not adapted. If all foods contain more or less harmful molecules, then excluding one of them will not change much, and so the study will not give the best results. With Genefit Nutrition, it was possible to approach the problem the other way around. Instead of trying to exclude a food suspected of generating health problems, the idea was to start from scratch, with the basics of nutrition, in applying a chimpanzee-like diet, excluding all forms of processing, and so getting rid of all possible sources of artificial harmful molecules at once.

Once geneticists understand how the human genome really operates in all its details we will have all the answers we need regarding our question of genetic adaptation. There will be no more doubt about what type of diet to apply to enjoy a healthy and long-lasting life. Unfortunately, we are far from understanding the human genome. The complexity of DNA, with at least thirty-five thousand genes interacting with each other in a still mysterious way, leaves us a rather slim chance of finding answers about humans' optimal diet. But we don't have to wait for connections to be made between properties of our DNA and our daily foods. Darwin, after all, didn't need genetics to write *The Origin of Species* and genetics confirmed his discoveries a century later. With Genefit Nutrition, we are currently in a similar situation. Like Darwin, the best we can do is rely on empirical evidence.

Genefit Nutrition is primarily based on empirical evidence. Unlike other "paleo-diets," it is not just a theory of human evolution that has led to conclusions about what to eat. It is based primarily on meticulous observations over the years, in comparing how the body reacts in the most subtle ways when switching between the two different food environments: traditional processed foods and exclusively unprocessed foods. The advantage of relying on empirical evidence is that when new discoveries are made concerning our evolutionary past, we don't have to change our diet because the previous one has been proven to be inaccurate or unsafe. Present-day observation and empirical evidence are by far the most reliable tools when it comes to finding answers to our questions. But, at the same time, information gathered from our evolutionary history, such as archaeological records, can give us hints, directions, and confirmations.

The large-scale experiment that led to Genefit Nutrition is unique in the world. No other study on the subject has ever been so far reaching. Decades ago, this research started with one question: Can human beings live a healthier life with the total exclusion of food processing? In view of the conclusive results we observed, the answer is undoubtedly yes.

Since experimentation started, thousands of people have chosen to apply a way of eating that totally excludes processed foods and uses the nutritional instinct as their exclusive guide. Some have chosen to remain on it to this day. People of all ages, from all over the world, have been practicing Genefit Nutrition, or a similar method of using the nutritional instinct, for periods of time ranging from a few days to a lifetime. Observations have been gathered over three consecutive generations. Children have grown up on this way of eating without deficiencies, tooth decay, or other problems that might be expected to result from an inadequate diet. Experience not only showed that it is possible to live an entire life on a diet excluding food processing, but also that many pathological conditions improved dramatically when switching to such a diet. Genefit Nutrition gets rid of all potential nutritional disturbance factors at once. With the absence of abnormal and unnatural molecules in the bloodstream and the brain, past and present experimentation brought surprising insights about how the body, brain, and nervous system work under truly natural eating conditions.

Genefit Nutrition sets new standards of nutrition with a *tabula rasa* of food processing. It takes advantage of the extraordinary legacy the earliest humans, our ancestors, left us. It is ancient wisdom for a modern world, which comes as a gift for the well being of present and future generations.

THREE

The Human Nutritional Instinct

Instinct: "A natural impulse or propensity that incites animals, including man, to the actions that are essential to their existence, preservation and development . . . a propensity prior to experience and independent of instruction."

Webster Universal 1999

"INSTINCTS," FOR VARIOUS REASONS, are not in vogue at this time. Many consider them to be "base," vile . . . or worse. Others deny their existence. Sigmund Freud, who postulated an unpopular "death instinct," no doubt had something to do with it. We currently prefer other explanations for why we do what we do. We prefer to say it is our personality, or our education, or some other cause that makes us act in one way or another. But instinct is for the birds, the bees, and the beaver — not for us. It is generally assumed that if instinct does in fact exist in humans, it is so weak as to be negligible.

In the early 1980s, a book by Nobel Prize winner E.O. Wilson titled *Sociobiology* went against the popular current. The book is a summary of observations and studies of behavioral instinctive patterns in many species, including human beings. Acclaimed by some, the final chapter about human instinctive behavior was severely attacked by detractors who didn't want to see human beings as instinct-driven animals. Scientific opinion remains susceptible to the influence of popular beliefs, in spite of constant attempts to keep it purely objective. Now, years after, *Sociobiology* laid the groundwork for the creation of a new field of science known as evolutionary psychology. The field of evolutionary psychology considers the likelihood that our mind has been shaped by evolution and that even the way we reason follows similar instinctive patterns across cultures. In fact, eminent evolutionary psychologists such as Steve Pinker have concluded that language itself is an instinct. Although different types of languages exist throughout the world, the impulse to speak in babies is instinctive and universal. According to Pinker, the basis of grammar appears to be innate, as if all languages in the world build upon the same instinctive canvas. And yet language is the foundation of culture — of any culture. A human society without language would present a quite different picture. Should we then conclude that instincts are the foundations our culture is built on?

Surely, instincts are the obvious and sometimes hidden driving forces in our societies. Recent developments in new scientific fields makes informed judgment concerning the limit between acquired behavior and instinctive behavior extremely blurry. Is a bird aware of its own instincts, or are they so built-in that they escape its consciousness? We, too, probably experience a sort of instinct blindness, making it difficult to be aware of our own instincts as being instincts. Thanks to our analytic intelligence, we have the unique ability to reflect on our own instincts. As we consider the instinctual phenomenon in ourselves, we may conclude that humans, instead of being the least instinctively driven animals, have in fact the most complex network of instincts, giving us the impression that we enjoy total freedom.

In fact, because of our genetic heritage, human beings are in many ways similar to animals, particularly the higher vertebrates. Newborn babies particularly resemble animals in their behaviors. They act on feelings (or "senses," or "instinct") alone. No rules, no principles, no recipes guide them until they grow older. The higher brain functions, once they develop, may repress or deviate from the earlier ones, but they are not eliminated. So, the "animal-like" behaviors of the human infant remain present — although perhaps held in check — in the adult.

One of the very first things a newborn baby wants to do is eat. Under natural circumstances, he or she cries for food, and the mother responds by offering her breast. This behavior can be observed in cats, dogs, horses, and all other mammals. And almost without exception animal mothers are able and willing to provide enough milk for their baby's needs. Should the same be true for human babies?

Interestingly, within hours of birth, human babies have been seen to be able to eat and digest fresh mango, banana, papaya, and a variety of other foods they were attracted to and that their mothers either pre-masticated or provided whole to suck upon. Babies will, in fact, frequently abandon the breast and clamor for fruit the mother is eating, the odor of which has reached them while nursing.

How does this come about? How does an animal — or a human baby — know what it needs to eat? To put it another way, does an animal or baby *know* what it needs at all? Or is it a case of "Mama knows best"? As far as animals are concerned, the obvious answer would be that the animal doesn't really *know* what's good for it. It just eats whatever is appealing, whatever has an attractive smell and taste. In order to explore this phenomenon, we propose an experiment the reader can easily try with a dog. If you don't own a dog, perhaps you can borrow one. For this experiment, don't fill Fido's bowl with dog biscuits, canned dog food, or any other mixture or commercial product. Offer him a banana. Dogs sometimes like bananas, and this *sometimes* is the central point of our experiment. If Fido's body isn't ready for a banana at this time, he'll turn away from it. Try again later, or give him a raw carrot, or fresh strawberries, or any other fresh, unprocessed fruit or vegetable. There is a good chance, however, that Fido will go for the banana. Feed it to him bite by bite. If he finishes the first banana, give him another one and keep going for as long as he wants it. At some point, he'll eat no more. He'll turn away. Even if Fido tries to keep eating bananas to please you, he can't. As you can observe, the piece of banana will fall out of his mouth, instinctively pushed out by his tongue. Soon his head will turn away and there is nothing in the world that can make Fido swallow any more banana after this point.

This is exactly what a baby who is on Genefit will do if offered an unprocessed food his or her body doesn't want. But Fido is more fortunate than babies on a traditional diet, because no one ever declared that bananas were good for dogs — whereas bananas, by tradition if not by prescription, are thought to be good for babies.

Once Fido has stopped responding to the banana offerings, you might think he is no longer hungry or that his stomach is full. Now, let's put this hypothesis to the test and offer him a piece of raw meat. If he eats it, he is still hungry, even though he is no longer hungry for bananas. This very simple experiment unveils one of the most fundamental phenomena nutritional science has substantially neglected to explore. Fido has an "alliesthesial taste barrier," which prevents him from eating a specific food he no longer needs. Michel Cabanac, a Canadian researcher, was the first to give this phenomenon a scientific name. He coined the word *alliesthesia* to describe that a given stimulus can arouse pleasure or displeasure according to the inner state of the body.

A food tastes and smells good when the body needs it, and the taste turns bad when the body doesn't need it anymore. It is a biochemical reaction of the body, allowing a very precise food intake regulation. Every one of us once knew about it, because when we were babies it was our guide to what we wanted, which was exactly the same as what we needed. This phenomenon permits every animal of every species to *know*, without recourse to dietetic theory, precisely what it needs to eat, and how much. It is an organismic message that says, unequivocally, when something good-tasting turns into something bad-tasting, I have had all I need. When people eat naturally, they regain this instinctive sense. This is how every species of living organism *knows* what it needs to survive. It eats what smells or tastes good, and turns away from what smells or tastes bad. When it has fulfilled its need for one particular food, it has also fulfilled its want, and turns away. This is what Fido did with the bananas and this is a capacity you will rediscover for yourself, if you carry out further experiments in this book.

The human senses of smell and taste would provide an infallible guide as to what types and amounts of food our bodies require, but for one thing: human "intelligence." Human beings are the only living species to feed on the milk of another species, to mix and season, to cultivate grains and other plant types, and above all, cook their foods. But the alliesthesial taste barrier does not occur with any food that is not in a strictly unprocessed state. This unfortunate and demonstrable fact has profound implications for our well-being.

> When an animal eats, it acts like a computer; that is, the most sophisticated kind of computer, that could choose the best quality foods in the right amounts, better than an expert dietician ever could. Conversely, man is like a broken-down computer, which compels him to eat anything, anyhow, and

which sometimes leads him to obesity or alcoholism (flaws that never occur with animals in a natural condition) . . . .

Food, according to its chemical composition, is broken down into fats (glycerides), sugars (saccharides), and proteins (nitrogenous food such as eggs, grains, meat, and fish). . . .

When it makes its choice, an animal is able to pick the foods it needs to balance input against output accurately from the relevant nutrients. An American, Professor Richter, was the first to demonstrate that rats were remarkably able when it came to selecting from a range of foods the appropriate amounts of protein, vitamins, and mineral salts necessary for their continued health. Even better, rats can change their minds, when their internal balance is experimentally tampered with. In this way, rats automatically increase their salt intake after removal of their adrenal glands; they will eat fats over sugars once they have been turned into diabetics; they select whatever vitamin they happen to be deficient in. . . . "This is most striking in chickens. . . . Chickens pick the amount and kind of food they require solely on the basis of the needs of the egg they lay daily. . . .

"When producing egg white, the chicken only eats whole, high-protein food. When the egg is taking up water, the hen drinks plentifully. Finally, when the shell is forming, the hen goes for calcium. One might imagine that that was due to circadian rhythm. Not so at all, since when chickens are raised from birth in constant light — that is, when they don't experience nighttime — their eating cycles remain unchanged. Further proof would be contributed from chickens that do not or no longer lay, or even from roosters. In the foregoing, there is no staggered intake of protein, calcium, or water. What's more, given that fowl can make up for the loss (incurred through laying its eggs, a case in point) by relevantly adjusting the quality of their food, they can also balance their diet — which Man can't do" ("Marching orders straight from the organs," *Science et Vie* [*Science and Life*] no. 729, June 1978).

The above excerpt points out the biggest misunderstanding science has faced when studying a potential nutritional instinct in humans. Several studies have been conducted to reveal the existence of such an instinct, but they failed to do so because no discernment was made between processed food altered by man's hand and unprocessed food as it can be found in nature. Erroneous conclusions have been drawn because of the incapacity of the nutritional instinct to recognize the chemical structure of modified food. So, it has been universally concluded that humans have lost their nutritional instinct.

PART TWO

Rediscover Your Nutritional Instinct

WE CHOSE TO ORGANIZE THIS BOOK in a way that permits readers to discover the fundamental principles of Genefit Nutrition, in the same way they were discovered. You will reproduce for yourself the actual experiments that have led to this extraordinary way of eating. Every experiment comes with an explanation and interpretation of corresponding phenomena. You will come to understand experientially how your own nutritional instinct works and how you can reach perfect nutritional balance. If you actually perform these experiments, you can test the validity of our claims about the nutritional instinct, and understand them more clearly than words alone would permit. The simple tasting and smelling experiments described in the following chapters can be reproduced by anyone of any age.

FOUR

Eating Pleasure as Guide

EXPERIMENT 1

Buy one or two pineapples (organic strongly recommended). It is important that the fruit has not been frozen, ground, cooked, treated, or otherwise modified in any way. It has to be in its original state. Since so much processing is applied that may not be evident, we suggest the use of exclusively fresh pineapples or other fruit or vegetables that can readily be recognized as such. This experiment can also be done for instance with organic cabbage, kiwi, fresh figs. For more "mild-tasting" foods the body might need some more training or fine-tuning, but don't worry, together, we'll get there.

To obtain the best possible results, it is better to do this experiment in the morning on an empty stomach. Begin to eat the pineapple by itself, in its natural state, without sugar or any other embellishment. Most people will experience a sweet and pleasant taste during the first few bites. Pay attention to the perception of the taste during the whole experiment. After eating a certain quantity, you will notice that the taste changes. It goes from sweet and pleasant to acidic, unpleasant, and even painful, like a burning sensation in the mouth or on your lips. At this point, if you keep eating, your lips may start to bleed! There is no way to influence the change of taste by will or by thought. Even if you think to yourself, "the pineapple is still sweet," it will start to burn anyway. This result demonstrates that the person performing the experiment does not consciously induce the change of perception. Of course, the pineapple hasn't changed either. Only the body's needs have changed. As long as there is a need for the nutrients contained in the pineapple, the taste is pleasant. When those needs are met, the perception of the taste becomes unpleasant or painful.

EATING PLEASURE has always been the main motivation for the culinary arts. There is no doubt that pleasure occupies a central place in our lives. It is eating pleasure that makes us go to distant restaurants. It is also pleasure that moves us to spend time — sometimes a lot of time —

preparing our food. And similarly, it is pleasure that moves us to continually seek new and better recipes. There is indeed a very good reason for this. Somewhere in our deep unconscious mind, we have an equation inherited from the animal world: *eating pleasure = survival*. In the wild, it is thanks to the nutritional instinct that an animal finds the foods and nutrients needed, not only to achieve top fitness, but to stay alive. And how does this instinct express itself? The answer is: through the amount of eating pleasure. When we use our nutritional instinct correctly, eating pleasure is the direct consequence of the fulfillment of our nutritional needs. The more an animal experiences eating pleasure, the better it follows its nutritional instinct, the better it covers its nutritional needs, and so maximizes its chances of survival. For the subconscious, eating pleasure is the confirmation of dietary balance; it is proof of health.

Now, if we reverse that equation, we obtain: *lack of pleasure = fear of death*. An animal that is unable to stay healthy because it is malnourished might not survive. This means that for us, at least a certain quantity of daily eating pleasure is mandatory to attain peace of mind. The constant quest for eating pleasure is driven by the unconscious mind because a lack of eating pleasure means fear of death, and a state of fear is an uncomfortable state to be in. This is why most diets fail: lack of eating pleasure. One might follow a diet to obtain better health, but since diets are mainly based on restrictions, they generate profound anxieties or even panic, making it impossible to resist cravings, causing the return to former dietary habits.

Genefit Nutrition is probably the only "diet" in which maximizing eating pleasure is the major rule. It is actually even more than a rule; it is an obligation, because within the boundaries of an unprocessed food supply, eating pleasure is your guarantee for health and nutritional balance. With Genefit, you will be "forced" to have fun while eating because the more eating pleasure you have, the more you will find yourself on the path toward the results you want.

Of course, you might have concerns about how to find eating pleasure with some raw carrots and a few fruits. It is important to remember that nature provides *all* the conditions for every animal to attain inner quietness through high levels of eating pleasure. Since the equation *eating pleasure = survival* results from evolution within an unprocessed food environment, nature has also made available the conditions and the tools to feel comfortable with it. All animals have lived on unprocessed raw food since the beginning of time. When they find the food they need, they do not seem to express any particular panic or fear of death because of a lack of pleasure. Chimpanzees taking a nap after a copious lunch under a fruit tree do not seem to lack eating pleasure. The whole picture resembles more a feeling of fulfillment — a very deep quietness. In animals, taste buds and related brains centers are perfectly adapted to unprocessed foods so they provide enough eating pleasure to live comfortably without processing. Why should it then be different for humans?

Actually, it is different for humans, but not because of nature. Processed food leads to constant nutritional overloads of certain nutrients, such as carbohydrates, fats, and proteins. If we are perfectly honest, most of us will report that we often have a tendency to eat outside our body's real needs. Isn't that one of the main purposes of culinary arts? Food processing makes food taste "better" than nature. At least that is what is universally believed. Food processing tricks the nutritional instinct, so one is able to eat even if there is no need. The resulting biochemical imbalance tends to reduce eating pleasure with food that remains unprocessed. With unprocessed food the level of eating pleasure is directly proportional to the body's needs. Now, when the body is already overloaded or subject to biochemical imbalance because of processed food, it never fully needs the nutrients from unprocessed foods — the foods where the nutritional instinct works properly. As a result, the maximum eating pleasure available from unprocessed food can't be experienced initially.

When you first start applying Genefit Nutrition, you will not experience the natural levels of eating pleasure. Only when the body is clear of daily overloads and the bloodstream clear of abnormal molecules caused by food processing, will full eating pleasure return. This change will take a few days to a week. People on Genefit for a couple of weeks report that eating pleasure is much higher than it was with traditional food. Food is so universally processed, people don't naturally endure the first ascetic days of a purely unprocessed food diet, so the image of unprocessed food being unpleasurable persists. But this is not the case at all for those who make it through the first few days.

Nonetheless, if eating pleasure is something we enjoy lightly, it is in reality more than simple fun. Too often, we have considered eating pleasure a luxury, something without purpose or theoretical value. For most people, the pleasure of eating is just pure fun, something we may take or leave as we wish. In the eyes of a behaviorist, things are a little different. For the behaviorist, pleasure is the aim or motivation that causes an animal to move or travel for its own good. In the wild, pleasure always serves a purpose. Even young cats playing with each other are indeed practicing for future hunting, probably without even realizing it; they are simply practicing with the pleasure of playing. Pleasure and displeasure are the very roots of animal and human psychology, because they are so closely related to survival. For a baby, the pleasure of eating is as built-in or innate as the drive to eat itself. Pleasure is clearly instinct related. Pleasure never exists without some attendant benefit, in the same way an instinct never exists without a purpose. In fact, pleasure never exists without the purpose of the instinct to which it is related; otherwise, it would be a waste of energy. In the natural world, energy is precious and wasting it produces a competitive disadvantage.

The instinct to eat, like every other instinct, has a clear purpose. If we draw a rough diagram of an instinct, it will look like this:

Impulse or drive ▶ pleasure or satisfaction ▶ purpose or survival benefit

And in the case of nutrition, in particular, we obtain something like this:

Impulse to eat ▶ pleasure of eating ▶ nourishment of the body

As we can see, pleasure makes sense as long as it exists within a purpose. In the case of nutrition, if everything goes well, pleasure finds its natural position by serving the true needs of the body. The diagram above is the perfect picture of nutrition: hunger triggers the impulse to eat, and while the impulse is assuaged, pleasure is involved. In the end, the primary impulse reaches its goal, which is to nourish the body. It is important to see that as long as pleasure is connected to a purpose, it is naturally appropriate for it to be completely guilt free, since it serves one's health, and therefore promotes the preservation of life.

Every time we eat outside our body's true needs, or we eat food that is not natural, somewhere in the back of our minds there is a little feeling of guilt, a voice that says, "I know I shouldn't eat that. It isn't good for me, but what the hell . . ."

Guilt is generally experienced at two different levels:

1. The first is a cultural level. Guilt may be experienced when rules or laws of a specific religious, cultural, or social context are broken. Such feelings of guilt can change from country to country, or region to region, or even from family to family. However, this is a superficial form of guilt that can easily be suppressed.
2. The second level of guilt is innate or built-in. It is the guilt one experiences when intentionally breaking laws of nature inherent to the order of life. This type of guilt is generated from deep down in the subconscious and is impossible to suppress. Even if repressed, it will still persist.

The feeling of guilt felt when overeating or eating unhealthy food is, to a certain extent, innate. It originates directly from a conflict with the preservation instinct: eating something that can be harmful is against life, and overeating is, in the long run, harmful. The only way to eat without experiencing any guilt at all, even deep down in our subconscious, is to eat according to our body's real needs, in terms of both quality and quantity. But how do we do that? How do we know for sure what is needed or appropriate?

Of course, one can count calories, institute restrictions, buy vitamin pills, etc., but this is not what Genefit Nutrition is all about. Our method is much more efficient and accurate. With Genefit, food is as natural as it gets, and the intake is regulated by the nutritional instinct — function created by life itself.

In our first experiment, we came in contact with the phenomenon of *gustatory alliesthesia*, which is the change of perception in taste while eating. In a strictly unprocessed food environment, pleasure does not obey one's will. It is the body itself in relation with the food that releases, or allows, eating pleasure. The conscious mind has no control over the process. Within the alliesthesial guidance, pleasure of eating is totally guilt free, because you listen to your own body's wisdom, and therefore to related laws of nature which have been determined by the harsh con-

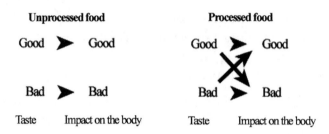

FIGURE 4. The function of taste in unprocessed and processed food environments.

ditions of natural selection. As long as gustatory alliesthesia is working — and we will later define precisely when it is and when it is not — overeating is virtually impossible. Eating is truly done in accordance with the body's needs.

By using your nutritional instinct, you will enjoy an innocent and playful approach toward food and dietary issues. You will be able to eat in a carefree frame of mind, because the more pleasure you experience while eating a food, the better it is for your body. You will no longer say to yourself: "I shouldn't have eaten that. It isn't good for my health or figure." You will no longer experience the conflict between the pleasure of eating and guilt, because the food you just ate is known to be unhealthy, or because you overate.

The implications of Experiment 1 are surprisingly far reaching. In an unprocessed food environment, gluttony does not exist. Gluttony is a human invention that followed the rise of the culinary arts. Chocolate, for example, offers no safety net against overeating. On the other hand, the cacao fruit, which is nature's original chocolate, actually has a taste that is very close to its processed cousin when the body needs it and a fiercely unpleasant one when the body has fulfilled its needs. The terribly bitter sensation is so strong that it is impossible to overcome. Thus, chocolate addiction does not exist with cacao fruit. As long as one eats in accordance with his or her body's needs, even large quantities can, by definition, never be considered gluttony.

The gustatory alliesthesia you have experienced with Experiment 1 is only the first step into the world of Genefit Nutrition. As we will see in the following experiments, there are many other expressions of the nutritional instinct. Gustatory alliesthesia is the primary mechanism that regulates food intake. With this built-in function, it has never been so easy to eat the exact quantity your body needs. Within the limits of a strictly unprocessed food supply, there is no need to apply intellectual limitations. Gustatory alliesthesia provides many obvious advantages over intellectual approaches. In fact, the nutritional instinct is as capable of solving math problems as the intellect is of solving dietary problems. Putting each tool in its respective place, corresponding to its natural function, is the right way to go. Trying to set up our diet with our intellect is a little bit like using a screwdriver as a hammer; even if it somehow works, it wasn't made for that. So much for home improvement advice . . .

For the sake of clarity, the gustatory alliesthesia experience has been split into four distinct phases, which one goes through during consumption of a given food:

Ecstatic phase: This phase gives maximum eating pleasure and occurs when the body needs all the nutrients in a given food. Because the body is fully in sync with the food, the level of eating pleasure experienced is much greater than the level one normally experiences with a traditional diet. The quality of taste is so different that it exceeds any representation you can possibly have. Eating a food in the ecstatic phase provides new flavors unknown to people who have never been on Genefit. For example, seeded, nonhybridized grapes taste better than the most delicious jam pancake or ice sorbet you have ever eaten. Ecstatic phases can never be experienced while on a traditional diet, because of nutritional overloads and the impact of abnormal molecules on the metabolism. After an adjustment period, as soon as the body goes back to its original way of functioning thanks to the cleansing effect of Genefit Nutrition, those ecstatic phases become possible.

Pleasant phase: This phase gives some eating pleasure and occurs when the body needs only some of the nutrients in a given food. In this phase, the product is still beneficial to the body. This is typically the phase you experience when you simply enjoy eating grapes, for example. While being on a traditional processed diet, most people's gustative representation of the taste of a delicious fruit lies in this phase. This is also the highest phase one is able to experience if Genefit is not applied correctly.

Unpleasant phase: This phase occurs when the body signals that some nutrients are unwanted or harmful. If you eat your grapes while in this phase, you may find yourself spitting out the seeds and skin. Or you may think the grapes are bad because they don't have a pleasant taste. Spitting out skin and seeds is a form of slight processing, where the intellect is used to trick the instinct, in order to be able to eat more than your body actually needs.

Painful phase: This is the strongest stop signal the body can give. Constantly eating until the painful phase may, in the long run, be painful, not only to your mouth, but to your whole body. The painful phase is not always literally painful. It can also take the form of an impression of swallowing difficulty, a change of consistency, or it may produce a sensation of having a coating on your teeth. In general, this stage takes the form of an extreme unpleasantness in taste or consistency.

During the consumption of a given food, one goes from the ecstatic phase, if your body really needs it, all the way to the painful phase, if you insist on eating beyond your body's needs. The "taste curve" that occurs during the consumption of a given food is the real-time report of the biochemical state of the body and its needs. This sensory information resembles reports from a database, updated with every bite you take.

Besides providing an extremely high level of eating pleasure, the ecstatic phase also produces a slight state of euphoria. Constantly eating in the ecstatic phase provides a permanent natural high. An interesting conclusion can be drawn from this observation: if a more or less permanent state of euphoria is the natural state for human beings to be in, the loss of it is intuitively experienced as abnormal or unnatural. Most individuals will have a strong drive to seek this state, but since the ecstatic phases do not occur when food is processed, they have a tendency to look for it in the wrong places, for instance, by using recreational drugs. Here, we are talking about legal drugs, such as alcohol, caffeine, and antidepressants, as well as illegal drugs. We have distanced ourselves too much from a natural way of eating to remember that eating unprocessed

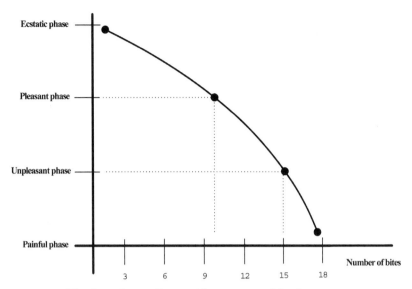

FIGURE 5. The four phases of taste with unprocessed foods.

food in ecstatic phases produces continuing euphoric states. The state of euphoria provided by ecstatic phases comes without the incapacity of focusing, mental unavailability, or any other secondary unhealthy effects known from drugs. Not only does the ecstatic phase have no negative effect on health, it is the confirmation that one is on the path of optimal fitness. Of course, food alone will not make you fully happy; there are many other factors involved. But, if you get a chance to experience these phenomena yourself, you will see that ecstatic phases offer an interesting setting in which to boost your "happy meter" higher than usual.

There is one more body signal that regulates the intake quantity of food that needs to be taken into consideration: *repletion*. Repletion is the medical term for a sensation of pressure in the stomach — a sensation of fullness. In an unprocessed food environment, this sensation of fullness has nothing to do with the quantity one eats. Repletion can occur with very minimal quantities — after just one or two bites. On the other hand, it is possible not to feel any pressure in the stomach, even when large quantities are eaten. Repletion is a part of the human nutritional instinct, but is not necessarily related to the physical volume of the stomach. Repletion is a warning signal occurring when the digestive capacity of the body is about to be exceeded. As you will experience, it is sometimes possible to obtain a sensation of fullness even before the change of taste has occurred. There are two main reasons for this:

1. The first is the quality of the food supply. Hybridized and artificially selected plant products (fruits and vegetables) do not exactly suit our genetic makeup. In this case, our instinctive computer gets information through the taste buds that is somewhat blurry. Sometimes the sensation of fullness occurs to avoid overeating. Experiencing fullness with wild, nonhybridized foods is extremely rare.
2. The second is the biochemical state of the body. The longer you practice Genefit Nutrition, the less you will experience the sensation of fullness. Repletion is mainly regulating the detoxification processes. As the body cleans itself with unprocessed food, the internal biochemical balance adjusts, and gustatory alliesthesia is better able to take exclusive control of your food intake.

In summary, there are two distinct instinctive signals or "stops" that may occur while eating a given food. The first one is a change of taste, and the second is repletion. To ensure optimal dietary balance and well-being, it is important to listen to whichever comes first.

FIVE

The Instinctively Balanced Diet

Repeat Experiment 1 with the same food for several mornings. You will notice a difference in the quantities you will be able to consume before the change in taste occurs. Your body's needs change from day to day — even within the day. Your instinct will adjust your food intake to what is needed at any given time.

FEW PEOPLE KNOWLEDGEABLE in matters of nutrition would dispute the following statements. Yet, they contain a fundamental error. Can you spot it?

The list of raw materials we need from our environment is a long one, and the list is largely what nutrition is all about. We need calcium ions, phosphorous ions, sodium ions, potassium ions, chloride ions, magnesium ions, ferric or ferrous ions, zinc ions, manganese ions, copper ions, cobalt ions, molybdenum ions, iodine, leucine, isoleucine, valine, methionine, theonine, phenylalanine, some form of Vitamin A, some form of Vitamin D, some form of Vitamin E, some form of Vitamin K, Vitamin C, thiamine, riboflavin, pantothenate, niacinamide, biotin, folic acid, pyridoxine, and Vitamin B12.

Unbelievable as it may seem, we need all of these elements in about the right amounts every day (or every two days) or we suffer. Furthermore, there is excellent evidence that all of the elements listed constitute absolute needs. If we fail to get them and run out of our reserves, we will surely die. It gives one an odd feeling to realize that our very existence depends every day on the practical solution of an equation with 40 or more variables (Quoted by Schultz & Myers in *Metabolic Aspects of Health*, Discovery Press, Kentfield, 1979).

Did you spot it — the "minimum daily requirement" concept? Commonly found on the labels of vitamin bottles, cereal boxes, and bread packages, it underlies the precept of the "apple a day" or the morning dose of orange juice. If such things were necessary in our distant past, the human race would not have survived long enough to become human. There were no supermarkets in the jungle; such calculated balancing acts would have been impossible. But, even today, if we really take a closer look at all our acquired scientific knowledge and modern technology, there is still no way to determine precisely what quantity of each nutrient is needed by a given individual's body at a given moment. The chemical processes involved inside the body are too complex for our analytic means. Daily minimum requirements are only based on averages. They can't tell us specifically what each individual needs at any given time. Dietetic recommendations are simplifications and approximations of what is currently believed to be a balanced diet. For now, these are the best nutritional guidelines science has to offer. As a result, when somebody tells us, "Eat a balanced diet; it is your best guarantee for good health," it is impossible to know exactly what this means. But, in order to achieve optimal health, or to recover it during illness, a very precise intake regulation is the first necessary step.

The following example shows how misleading it can be to base a diet on averages and minimum requirements. Thirty years ago, the difference between unsaturated fats and saturated fats was unknown. Soon after their discovery, unsaturated fats were recognized as essential for the prevention of cancer. Formerly, prescriptions for an ideal diet were devised without specific reference to unsaturated fats. However, we now know that low-fat diets that exclude them completely for long periods of time are very dangerous. Unsaturated fats are part of the so-called daily minimum requirements. Since the distinction has been made between what are sometimes called "bad fats" and "good fats," dieticians have revised the concept of an optimal diet, which means that all the former prescriptions for what was believed to be a healthy diet were inaccurate. People who trusted those prescriptions were misled. In order for someone to make infallible prescriptions, the nutritional theories behind those prescriptions need to be exempt from mistakes. But no health professional can, with a clear conscience, claim that the nutritional theories around nowadays are exempt from errors. Researchers are constantly discovering new nutrients and new factors involved in nutritional processes. We still have not mastered the chemical structure of a banana, for example. The proof is that if we take all the chemical elements we believe are in a banana and put them together, we still don't get something even close to a banana.

To make things even more complicated, combinations of nutrients are sometimes necessary for them to be assimilated by the body. For example, calcium is only assimilated by the body in the presence of vitamin D. Phosphate annuls calcium assimilation, so a very delicate balance between phosphate and vitamin D is necessary for the body to be able to take advantage of calcium. These are processes we know about, because calcium assimilation has been widely studied, but many other processes with other foods are far less well understood. Daily requirements in vitamin pills, for example, do not in any way follow the real-time fluctuations of daily natural needs. Some vitamins, such as vitamin E or D, can be dangerous when consumed in excessive quantities. They can accumulate in cells and create damage over time. Instead of thinking of the body as a high-performance engine that needs special and very specific care depending on the tasks that need to be done, it is not uncommon for dieticians to think of it as an oven into which we can put more or less whatever nutrients, as long as we get the approximate required doses of each. The body is too often thought of as a food burner that will cope with what is available and reject what is not needed. This view is simplistic and does not render an accurate picture of what is going on in the body at a molecular level.

As stated at the beginning of this chapter, it is true that unless a minimal amount of each and every nutrient our body requires is present, we will suffer from varying degrees of malnutrition. But the implication that there is a static, fixed minimum for human beings in general is wrong. The minimum amount of nutrients essential for health is not an average of the minimum amount that might be required over the course of several months or a year. Particularly in a therapeutic context, the minimum we require may greatly exceed the average requirements of a healthy body. In addition, the ingestion of a supposedly "necessary" nutrient may be toxic because it exceeds the body's requirement for it at that particular moment. A simple analogy will make it clear why this is so. Let us say we are going to build (or rebuild) not a body, but a house. So we are going to use not proteins, vitamins, amino acids, glucose, etc., but cement, rafters, wiring, pipes, windowpanes, and shingles. Let's say it's a hundred-day project. Now, it's mealtime (supply time) on the building site and here comes the lunch wagon (delivery truck), which is scheduled to come every day for a hundred days. In order to provide a "balanced diet" (of materials), logically, on the first and every succeeding day it will be carrying 1/100th of the cement requirement, one percent of the rafters, one percent of the wiring, etc. Shall we start building? How can we? How can we build when at each stage of construction we need all the material required at that stage? At the outset, we will need cement and reinforcing rods for the foundations. We will have no need for windowpanes at all. Many items not only can wait, but must wait. Construction has to proceed in a particular order or chaos will ensue.

When the body needs supplies for whatever it is building (or rebuilding) at a particular time, it needs the full amount of what is required, or it must leave the job unfinished. But just exactly what it does need, and when and how much, can only be determined by the individual, never by prescription. This propensity for individual variation becomes dramatically clear from observations of people on Genefit Nutrition eating their way to health. Their need for particular nutrients on any given day, or over a given period, may be so massive as to preclude all others, but once that need has been filled, it may not make itself felt again for many weeks. Nor are nutritional requirements ever the same for two different people on any given day, or for a given individual on succeeding days.

This claim does not result from speculation. In exceptional cases, often related to severe pathologies, instinct may lead a person to eat as many as 105 passion fruits at a sitting before the taste becomes unpleasant, and then to eat practically nothing but passion fruits again at the next meal, and the next, possibly for days on end. But then, abruptly, after some time, passion fruits will hold no more attraction, and the person will find herself making full meals of oranges and pineapples, or oysters, or spinach. Apparently, there was a tremendous deficiency in some area that was demanding priority. Once it was fulfilled, but not before, other requirements could make themselves felt. In such cases, the optimum intake quantity can be correctly determined only by following the body's sensory (instinctive) cues with native foods. Observations have always shown that when an unprocessed food is consumed instinctively, even in such large quantities, digestion was completely symptom free. The absence of symptoms during digestion in those cases also confirms the optimal functioning of the nutritional instinct.

Many people have come to us because they suffered from deficiencies, and have begun eating instinctively to quickly improve their conditions. A few years ago, Susie, who had a severe iron deficiency, spent some time with us. After testing all the foods available on our daily table, Susie chose the parsley — or should we say her body chose the parsley, because she wasn't very happy about her choice. Parsley is a food the body usually needs only in small quantities. When raw, most people experience a strong bitter taste after one or two bites. But, Susie didn't eat just a few leaves; she ate ten big bunches of parsley in one sitting! She described it as tasting like the best soup she ever ate. Her description must have been accurate; it would ordinarily be quite difficult for someone to eat such a quantity. The good news is that Susie's deficiency didn't last very long after she came to us. Parsley contains huge amounts of iron. Susie clearly did not choose this food by intellectual decision; otherwise, she would have chosen some delicious fruit. It was her body that guided her to the parsley and since her body needed iron, the taste remained amazingly good for the entire ten bunches.

A dietician could hardly be expected to prescribe ten bunches of parsley and, on the other hand, a patient couldn't be expected to be able to eat that much. In addition, even with the same diagnosis of iron deficiency, the body of another person might instinctively choose a totally different food. In this particular case, parsley might taste terribly bad. Experience indicates we can't just automatically prescribe huge amounts of parsley for everyone with the same diagnosis. There are far more chemical factors involved, which the body might use in one way or another during the consumption and digestion of parsley, than just iron itself.

Other people who came to us with various deficiencies were attracted, at first, to large quantities of specific foods, the consumption of which was accompanied by high levels of eating pleasure. This behavior is explained by the fact that their bodies were in a state of emergency. Replenishing deficiencies is the first step toward health. Under Genefit

Nutrition eating conditions, the connection between deficiencies and an extraordinary flavor is evidence of a little marvel at work — our nutritional instinct.

The notion of a "balanced" diet is a trap for many beginning practitioners of Genefit Nutrition. If you haven't been attracted to animal foods for a couple of months, you may tell yourself, "I haven't had any beef for so long, I'm sure I need some." Because of dietetic precepts, you may then proceed to eat some meat but take little if any pleasure in it and in fact, you may feel unwell. Any nutrient, and especially protein, eaten in excess can eventually have a harmful effect. Optimal health progresses with the precision of the intake regulation. In this regard, it seems that science can't give us a satisfying answer. At the same time, in a processed food environment, calculations and averages are the only tools left to maintain health, since there is no more alliesthesial guidance. Researchers, nutritionists, and dieticians do the best they can to cope with a situation that became problematic with the advent of food processing.

In an unprocessed food environment, on the other hand, we can rely on our nutritional instinct, like any other mammal. No one has ever seen a chimpanzee read a nutrient table to find out what to eat. Nonetheless, chimpanzees in the wild have achieved nutritional balance; otherwise, the species would have faced extinction some time ago. How did they do that? Occasionally, chimpanzees have been observed to turn toward green leaves that would appear to us to be less attractive than the various fruits available to them. Why? The answer is, because they follow instinctive attractions. At that particular time, those leaves were as attractive to them as their favorite fruits.

> Bitter principles and related constituents have been isolated from Vernonia amygdalina (Compositae), a plant ingested by wild chimpanzees sometimes suffering from parasite-related diseases in the Mahale Mountains National Park, Tanzania. These isolated constituents were the known sesquiterpene lactones (vernodalin, vernolide, hydroxyvernolide), and new stigmastane-type steroid glucosides (vernonioside A_1-A_4, for bitter-tasting constituents and vernonioside B_1-B_3, for nonbitter-related constituents). Antiparasitic activity tests of these constituents together with quantitative analyses of the major active constituents, vernodalin and vernonioside B_1, supported the hypothesis that Mahale chimpanzees control parasite-related diseases by

ingesting the pith of this plant, found to contain several steroid-related constituents. While the major active steroid-related constituents (vernonioside B_1 and its primary aglycone, vernoniol B_1) do not taste bitter themselves, it was hypothesized that the highly bitter constituents including vernodalin may play an important role as signals to the ingester guiding their choice of the appropriate plant, plant part, and possibly also as signals which help to control the amount of intake (K. Koshimizu , H. Ohigashi , M.A. Huffman, "Use of Vernonia amygdalina by wild chimpanzee: possible roles of its bitter and related constituents." Physiol Behav 1994 Dec;56(6):1209-16).

In addition to achieving nutritional balance, they apply instinctive self-medication. Chimpanzees with infectious or parasitic symptoms have been observed to be instinctively attracted to very specific plants — plants that are known to contain active chemicals against particular pathologies. The nutritional instinct of chimpanzees "knew" how to heal those pathologies long before humans performed medical research.

In 1989, I published the first detailed account of bitter pith chewing (Huffman and Seifu, 1989). This study was the first study to document sickness at the time of ingestion of a known medicinal plant by a chimpanzee in the wild and to follow the individual through to apparent recovery . . .

In the first case study, a female was observed to meticulously remove the leaves and outer bark from several young shoots and chewed on the exposed pith, sucking out only the extremly bitter juice. Within 24 hrs, she had fully recovered from a lack of appetite, malaise, and constipation. A similar incident was observed in December of 1991, and in this case an infection of the nematode worm Oe. stephanostomum dropped noticeably within 20 hours after the adult female chewed V. amygdalina pith. In both cases, the rate of recovery (20-24 hrs) was comparable to that of WaTongwe (African tribe) who traditionally use this plant as a treatment for similar symptoms. Indeed, among many African peoples this plant is prescribed treatment for stomachaches, and a number of parasite infections including bilharzia, malaria and pinworm (Michael A. Huffman, "The medicinal use of plants by chimpanzees in the wild," Primate Research Institute, Kyoto University, Inuyama [excerpts]).

Chimpanzees instinctively know how to use many different plants in the natural pharmacopoeia available in the rainforest. The capacity of chimpanzees to deal with the diversity of the rainforest, with its huge variety of plants, some extremely toxic, some beneficial, can only underline the precision with which the nutritional instinct works. With thousands and thousands of different plants available, an analytic approach would be hopelessly inadequate. The complexity of the therapeutic effects of natural plants is beyond the comprehension of humans, not to speak of a chimpanzee's brain. Ironically, a new scientific field called zoopharmacognosy studies the behavior of animals that use self-medication in order to discover new medicinal plants and possible new treatments for human diseases.

For an individual to be truly well nourished, his diet must, in a sense, be properly *imbalanced*. His current needs may require him to choose food that is quite different from the average requirements of the general population. Only his instinct, rather than prescriptions, can lead him to eat what he really needs and tell him when to stop eating.

If you have performed Experiment 2 for several days, you probably noticed that your daily consumption of a given food declined from day to day. Then, after a day or two without that food, your appetite for it probably reset itself. The reason for this change is simple. After a few days, or a few weeks, except in a few special cases, the body has covered its primary need for that food. As a result, your body begins to produce a taste barrier much earlier than it did in preceding days. If you wait a few days, your need for nutrients in that particular food will resurface to a certain extent.

It is important to follow your instinct during the entire process and allow your body to get the nutrients it craves, even if the quantities seem completely exaggerated. As long as your pineapples, for instance, are strictly unprocessed and you don't add sugar or anything else, you don't have to worry about your levels of consumption. Without the nutritional instinct you might not have thought of eating the necessary quantity of that specific food. Gustatory alliesthesia is a valuable guard against nutrient deficiencies — large and small.

After some time spent on Genefit Nutrition, these phenomena become amazingly clear. Dietary cycles become familiar, and after a few years, may even become seasonal. For example, every time a new fruit is in season there will be a strong attraction in the beginning of the season, and then after some time the level of eating pleasure will drop drastically as the body covers its needs. In exceptional cases, we have observed people eating a specific fruit daily for several weeks, mainly during the body's reconstruction activity, without getting bored at all. As long as they needed the product, the taste was always delicious.

Phenomena such as gustatory alliesthesia also point out the importance of having a sufficient choice of foods available. It would not be much fun, and it would not be very safe, if we relied on only a few foods. For an average healthy person a minimum of ten varieties of fruits, ten varieties of vegetables, and ten high-protein or high-lipids-content foods will permit alternation between foods according to the nutritional instinct's "flavor of the day." The more different foods you have available, the better and easier it is for your body to find the shortest path to health.

Now, suppose we find ourselves in a strictly unprocessed food environment. Tastes of foods are changing and the nutritional instinct is working perfectly. How do we know for sure that gustatory pleasure corresponds to the body's true needs? This phenomenon might simply be random and have nothing to do with our real needs. If this were the case, one would become physically imbalanced in some way with Genefit Nutrition.

The growth of children under instinctive eating conditions is the most powerful confirmation of the good functioning of the human nutritional instinct — the direct link between sense of taste and the body's needs. In the past four decades, among all the families who started eating instinctively, we count two consecutive generations of children who grew up exclusively on unprocessed food. This large-scale experiment, triggered by the discovery of the human nutritional instinct, is truly unique in the world and a testament to the success of this way of eating.

One of those children is Jean, who is now twenty-eight years old and has eaten instinctively since birth. Jean and the many other children who grew up eating absolutely no processed food and using instinctive guidance are unique among the population of six billion people on earth. To our knowledge, no one else has practiced this program so precisely in recent history. These children constitute living proof that one can live and grow up healthily on Genefit Nutrition. None of them showed any signs of nutritional deficiencies during their entire growth period. Within the limits of an unprocessed food environment, they were permitted to

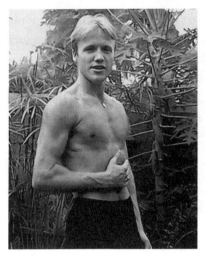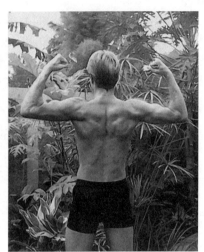

Jean on Genefit Nutrition since birth.

freely choose foods as their instincts directed them to. Not only have they shown no signs of nutritional deficiency, but they grew beautiful bodies, with perfectly developed muscles and bone structure.

As you can see, protein supply has not been a problem. Calcium supply has also been adequate, despite the fact that milk and dairy products are totally excluded from the diet. These children beautifully confirm our expectation that calcium can be found in sufficient quantity in unprocessed foods. Jean never took B12 supplements either, because animal products were part of his food palette. To date he has no cavities or any other sign of tooth decay. Unprocessed, unaltered foods evidently provide all the nutrients necessary for optimal growth, and the nutritional instinct is capable of guiding us to the right foods.

The observations gathered over two consecutive generations of children are a first milestone showing that it is possible to live in an unprocessed food environment over a long period of time and attain perfect health. Jean is still on Genefit Nutrition today and has no intention of changing his diet. Why should he?

Here, experimentation clearly demonstrates that the image of the struggling and rampant beast our modern societies have created when picturing our ancestors does not seem to reflect the reality of what really happened. The image of the hungry, violent, and sick caveman that we all have somewhere in our mind is more likely to be that of our ancestors who were already intensively cooking and were subjected to rheumatoid and arthritic problems, not because of rough living conditions, but because of the consumption of processed foods.

It has also been argued that the lifespan of our early ancestors did not exceed thirty-five years. Again, here, in the light of the evidence, we had to question our convictions. Interestingly, wild chimpanzees eating exclusively unprocessed foods and not applying any kind of human-imposed hygiene have a known lifespan of up to fifty-five years. So why should humans, who share a common ancestor, suddenly have their lifespan reduced to thirty-five years? Captive chimpanzees often develop serious health problems and die sooner than their wild cousins when they eat processed food regularly and in large quantities. The same could have happened to our ancestors. A shortening of the human lifespan is more likely to be the results of a processed, cooked food diet rather than the absence of it.

> Along with the new treatment of foods, there came an increased dependence on a few species of highly productive plants and animals that lent themselves to manipulation. This simplified human diets in comparison with those of the more eclectic hunter and gatherers and replaced a dependence on animal proteins with year-round ingestion of starches and carbohydrates, largely as milled and cooked cereals or tubers. Some of the most obvious effects of this change in diet were in the teeth where dental caries became a worldwide problem for the first time. With the spread of processed cooked foods came a reduction in the jaw musculature and the advent of overbite (overlapping of the upper incisor teeth with the lower ones).
>
> With agriculture, human populations became subject to entirely new health problems such as nutritional disease and periodic famine and starvation. (S. Jones , R. Martin , D. Pilbeam, "The Cambridge Encyclopedia of Human Evolution" [Cambridge University Press 1999], 2.7 p.378).

Until further laboratory work is done investigating the link between olfactory and gustatory receptors, the hypothalamus and other brain centers, and the metabolism, all we can do is rely on empirical evidence. Instinctively guided reversal of previously acquired deficiencies, deficiency-free growth of children under instinctive eating conditions, and fast recoveries in connection with a large consumption of a specific food are three powerful confirmations that the nutritional instinct really can tell us what to eat, how much to eat, and when to eat it.

SIX

What Is a "Natural" Food?

Buy one organic cabbage. Eat cabbage until a change of taste occurs, producing an unpleasant or burning sensation. Once you have reached this point, mix some olive oil or regular salad dressing with the cabbage. While you are eating, you will notice that you are now able to eat more cabbage without the unpleasant sensation. This experience shows that even if the body's needs are covered and the purpose of nutrition is reached, processing food allows us to push consumption further and eventually overeat. When food is unprocessed, what tastes good is good for the body and what tastes bad is unnecessary or harmful for the body. When food is processed, what tastes good can be bad for the body and what tastes bad can be, to a certain extent, good. This is the big contradiction in traditional food diets. As a result, intellectual knowledge and restrictions are necessary to stay healthy.

Note: Don't try to find a change of taste perception or an instinctive stop with processed food such as ice cream or chocolate. You might end up full, or eventually sick, but the taste won't change.

Take some fresh carrots, preferably organic. First, eat them raw in their unprocessed form until the taste changes (the taste of carrots becomes soapy when the body doesn't need them). Once you have reached this point, grind them. Eat the ground carrots until the taste becomes slightly unpleasant or simply boring. Now, take some of the ground carrots and juice them, and check the flavor of the carrot juice. It probably will taste passably good. Juicing allows you to totally overcome the original soapy taste you have previously experienced. Continue drinking the juice until the flavor again becomes boring, then put some sugar in the juice. From this point on, you are ready to drink as much juice as you want, but your actual body's needs were already covered with the change of taste occurring with the unprocessed carrots.

At each step of denaturing, you were probably able to gradually eat more and more carrots. Along all those steps, except for the unprocessed carrots, the taste no longer follows the real-time needs of the body. With the sugared juice, a change of taste becomes totally nonexistent.

EVERY SOCIETY has its popular nutritional traditions, habits, maxims, biases, and taboos. Culinary folklore is so pervasive that it affects even "scientific" nutritional maxims and practices. In one culture, physicians typically recommend against a specific food, because it is supposedly "hard to digest." In a different part of the world, physicians will prescribe it because "nothing is easier to digest."

Similarly, different countries thrive on different foods. Americans eat vast amounts of meat, wheat, and dairy products. Beans and corn are the staples in Mexico, rice and vegetables in China, potatoes in Germany, cabbage and herring in Russia, and so forth. Fortunately, the inhabitants of these countries do not limit themselves exclusively to these diets, but generally, they consider them to be "basic." As a premise, they assume that these staples are "natural" for the *Homo sapiens*, our species. Here, it must be emphasized that the nutritional habits of any culture are indeed precisely that: habits. They came into being the same way the language, music, and art of that culture arose: by circumstance and by chance. They are not necessarily "natural," i.e., native to humans the way plankton is native to whales.

The word "natural" has been perverted. Everyone knows what it means — and it means something different to different people. How do we define natural? Countless "natural" products are on the market, even in vending machines. Some are said to be more natural than others. So-called "organic" produce, for example, is thought to be more natural than foods grown with chemical fertilizers. It is also widely believed that *natural = good for you*. In order to avoid confusion, let us define "natural" as analogous to "primal" — unaffected by man's hand. If natural means directly and exclusively coming from nature, we have here a very simple definition that excludes much of what is commonly considered natural.

This point is fundamental, because for the millions of years of our evolutionary development, our predecessors did not possess, or at any rate did not use, enough cerebral cortex to change their food sources. They lived in an environment they could not transform. They might have found a cave to live in, but they couldn't build one. They could eat high-seas fish found dead on the beach, but they couldn't catch them in the ocean. They were dependent upon whatever their surroundings provided, the way they provided it. And this is where the word "natural" holds its true meaning.

They were also adapted to the foods in their environment. Had they not been, they would not have survived as a species until the time came when fire was mastered, the stone axe invented, or the discovery made that seeds could be planted in the earth. Until our ancestors developed some rudimentary technology and civilization, they chose their food the way animals do, the way our cousins the great apes do. Thanks to the automatic mechanisms of their biochemistry, what they needed was what they wanted. How, then, did we become so divorced from our nutritional instinct that we need to rely on laboratory analysis to know what is "good for us"?

The answer to this question lies in our inability to correctly evaluate any food that is not in its native, unprocessed state as it was over the hundreds of millions of years during which our biochemistry was evolving adaptively with it. When a food has been denatured — by cooking, for instance — it will not trigger an alliesthesial response. Once humans discovered how fire could be used for cooking, they were on a one-way trip to metabolic chaos and organic disharmony. They had tied a knot they couldn't undo, which we, their descendants, have rendered practically inextricable.

To acquire deeper understanding of this phenomenon, let us imagine a tribe of *Homo erectus* somewhere in Africa, say around 400,000 B.C. They are gathered near a fire, eating yams and other foods collected earlier in the day. The ones who are eating yams are those whose bodies need nutrients the yams contain (this is what makes them smell and taste good). Those who do not need yams are not attracted to them. Whatever they're eating, they are eating it raw, the way it came off a tree or out of the ground. It has never occurred to any of them to mix, grind, pound, heat, or do anything else to an attractive piece of food other than eat it.

One member of the group — call him "Onemug" — has eaten less than a fourth of a yam when the taste becomes unattractive. Carelessly he throws it down, and it rolls onto the edge of the fire, unnoticed. And there, it begins to bake. And it begins to smell. The smell reaches Onemug's nose, and it smells good. The smell is more fascinating than a yam ever smelled before. So Onemug follows his nose, and picks up the baked yam and begins to eat it. He can do so now, because the taste has become good again. The yam's molecular structure, modified by heat, no longer causes its taste to change from good to bad.

The following day, Onemug is hungry, but all the tribe has found to eat that day is yams. Thanks to the cooking, Onemug had been able to eat more yams than he actually needed, so his body is still overloaded with it. As a result, he finds the raw yam unattractive. But Onemug is a genius. He remembers that the hot yam from the fire was good, so he associates: *fire* + *yam* = *good*. On an impulse, he pushes a yam into the fire. Sure enough, an attractive odor eventually comes to his nose. He is able to eat the yam with a degree of pleasure until he's full. Of course, the other members of the tribe smell the cooked yam too, and begin to follow suit. So all of them begin to eat cooked yams, not just until their bodies have had their fill of the nutrients yams contain, but until their bellies have room for no more. The next day, because they don't need them, none of them are attracted to raw yams any longer.

This brings upon the tribe an unexpected change in the way it lives. Until now, yams in their natural state were, most of the time, delicious. Now, however, they have to be cooked or they can't be eaten. Instinct has to be tricked or it will stop the body from overloading itself with substances it doesn't need. Thus is birth given to the artifice of cooking. It is not yet an "art" in the sense of *haute cuisine*, but it must inevitably become one. For by disrupting the dynamic structure of instinctive taste for a food, cooking kills its flavor: each mouthful tastes just like the last. Since it will not trigger an alliesthesial response, it will not become unpalatable. But it will be boring, because the taste of cooked food does not vary.

Over the centuries, ways will be found to "enliven" it, to make it interesting and pleasurable to eat. Food in its original state will of itself be more pleasurable than any artifice can ever make it, but only if the body needs it. However, once the organism has become saturated with remnants of denatured food, which it can neither use nor eliminate, because biochemically it "doesn't know how," the senses of smell and taste themselves become denatured, and dulled. Thus must leaves, herbs, spices, ferments, oils, extracts, mixing, baking, roasting, basting, and boiling be called upon to provide some flavor where little remains. Today, scientists all over the world assume, along with everyone else, that cooking is perfectly "natural" for humans. The molecular effects of processing techniques on food, and the effects of processed food on the human body, have only recently become a subject for scientific inquiry. On many levels, the principles of Genefit Nutrition give us a clear understanding of the processes involved, and so provide us with the option to break the vicious circle of culinary art.

Onemug's story reminds us that cooking, and more generally food processing, are traps; once overloads and biochemical imbalance have been introduced by a processed food with which the nutritional instinct doesn't work, the attraction, and therefore the pleasure level, not only drops with the equivalent unprocessed food, but also with similar unprocessed ones. For example, a meal of roasted nuts will induce a protein overload. It will suppress attraction to all varieties of truly raw nuts and the eating pleasure they provide. Consuming a good amount of ice cream will induce an overload in artificial sugars and will suppress the natural attraction to all fruits and the eating pleasure they provide.

This phenomenon has a major consequence for anyone starting a diet involving instinctive guidance. As we saw in our first experiment, a certain amount of daily eating pleasure is mandatory to obtain profound satisfaction, and since processing gives easy access to eating pleasure despite overloads, one will always be drawn to continue eating the processed products until the natural pleasures that unprocessed food provides have been restored. What was a trap for humankind some hundred thousand years ago may still be, on a smaller scale, a trap for anybody starting on Genefit Nutrition A single, unnatural, sometimes even slightly processed food can put one's practice of Genefit Nutrition in jeopardy. The quality of your food supply is crucial: if correct, it is the foundation one can build on to obtain perfect dietary balance. When incorrect, it is the stone that makes one fall. In general, under Genefit eating conditions, the absence of high levels of eating pleasure is a signal of either a misuse of the nutritional instinct or a lack of quality in the food supply.

Being on Genefit Nutrition with an inadequate food supply is not being truly on Genefit Nutrition. It might be a raw food diet if food isn't heated, but it is not Genefit Nutrition as we define it. It is very important to point out that Genefit Nutrition at ninety-eight percent will not give you ninety-eight percent of the results. The last two percent will make *half* the difference. It is reasonable to expect that a diet that is almost perfectly healthy and contains only two percent of poisonous foods could be deadly. Similarly, in our experience, a diet is only two percent unnatural results in a large degradation in the expression of the nutritional instinct. If only one food goes outside the limits of our definition of natural food, you will no longer be able to rely on your nutritional instinct. The very precise change of taste will no longer reflect your body's true needs. The perfect dietary balance Genefit Nutrition provides will be disrupted.

Over three billion years of life history on Earth and no species thrived on processed foods — not until Onemug came along. As much as 99.9 percent of the entire evolution of life has been performed under unprocessed food conditions, with food the way nature provides it. If we really want to take advantage of the three billion years of wisdom written into our genes, we need to place Genefit Nutrition within the context in which it evolved, and this in a very precise manner.

It is very important to actually experience that the nutritional instinct doesn't work accurately with processed food, as you probably did in Experiment 3A or 3B. Otherwise, you might not understand why we put such importance on having a completely natural food supply. It is remarkable that such a simple change as grinding carrots could significantly alter the alliesthesial response. It is important to note that the absence of alliesthesial response strongly pleads for a genetic nonadaptation to even slightly processed food. And given the exacting requirements of our alliesthesial response, it is remarkable that people experimenting with pristine natural diets rediscovered it after it had been ignored for so long. Only the innateness of the nutritional instinct provides a plausible explanation for this phenomenon.

Another notion that Onemug's story brings to our attention is that there must have been signs or symptoms as a consequence of the repetitive consumption of the cooked yam. Our ancestors were certainly not genetically adapted to cooked yams, since they hadn't been exposed to them before. They were no more adapted to cooked yams than chimpanzees are today, and chimpanzees certainly develop human-like diseases when fed cooked foods. So, we can imagine that Onemug's first steps into culinary activities, however primitive, would eventually result in a collection of symptoms. They were probably minor ones in the beginning, such as poor digestion or headaches. When cooking became more sophisticated, more severe pathologies appeared, such as diabetes, pneumonia, and many more. Did Onemug's tribe conceive of the relationship between cause and effect? Did they consider the possibility that eating cooked yams resulted in symptoms and diseases? We don't know. Possibly, some individuals or even entire tribes did and others kept on cooking.

According to the archaeological records, some 360,000 years passed between the first known hearths and the widespread use of cooking. Why did it take so long? The time necessary to acquire the ability to master fire alone is not a satisfying consideration to explain such a long timeframe. One explanation could be that the relationship between cause and effect was made quickly. Perhaps seeing members of the tribe become sick was enough to keep our ancestors away from cooking, at least until 40,000 years ago. Another possibility could be that most tribes that were cooking extensively didn't survive at all, because of diseases or the competitive disadvantage it produced, leading to evolutionary dead ends. This would explain the famous bottleneck our species went through at some point in history:

> A worldwide research program has come up with astonishing evidence that humans have come so close to extinction in the past that it's surprising we're here at all.
>
> "We actually found that one single group of 55 chimpanzees in West Africa has twice the genetic variability of all humans," says Pascal Gagneux, an evolutionary biologist at the University of California at San Diego. "In other words, chimps who live in the same little group on the Ivory Coast are genetically more different from each other than you are from any human anywhere on the planet. . . . The family tree shows that the human branch has been pruned," Gagneux says. "Our ancestors lost much of their original variability."

"The amount of genetic variation that has accumulated in humans is just nowhere near compatible with the age of the species," says Bernard Wood, the Henry R. Luce Professor of Human Origins at George Washington University and an expert on human evolution. "That means you've got to come up with a hypothesis for an event that wiped out the vast majority of that variation." The most plausible explanation, he adds, is that at least once in our past, something caused the human population to drop drastically. When or how often that may have happened is anybody's guess. Possible culprits include disease, environmental disaster and conflict" ("We Dodged Extinction," Lee Dye for *ABC News*, Nov. 16 2001).

But then proceeding beyond speculations, symptoms can be observed every time a person who has been on Genefit Nutrition for some time eats food that has been processed. One of those symptoms is inflammatory pain. Inflammatory pain is no longer experienced when the body is nourished under strictly instinctive conditions. It might be difficult to believe, but this has been observed repeatedly. If one sustains a burn after being on an instinctive diet for some time, there may be pain for several minutes after the burn occurs, but then it stops. Long-lasting pain doesn't occur, as it does in people on a traditional diet of processed food. Under traditional eating conditions, pain can go on for hours after a burn or a cut, depending on its severity.

It is a popular belief that pain is a warning that something is wrong. If we put this belief in more mathematical terms, we may say that *pain = error*. This understanding is emphatically true when it comes to balance and well-being in nature; when somebody sustains a burn or an ape falls from a tree, we can safely assume that a mistake has been made. The first acute pain indicates that he has not been careful enough in the preservation of his body. Direct pain after an accident should not last more than a few minutes, just enough to inform the owner of the body that it is better not to make the same mistake again.

Experience had led us to conclude that long-lasting inflammatory pain is a result of abnormal molecules coming from food processing circulating in the bloodstream, since it doesn't exist under natural instinctive eating conditions. The presence itself of abnormal, artificial molecules in the bloodstream can, of course, also be considered an error, particularly since some of them have been proven to be harmful to the human body. This does rather suggest a problem — something that was not meant to be.

For people no longer subject to inflammatory pain thanks to Genefit Nutrition, eating even slightly heated nuts, fruit juices, or any other minor digression from the food's original state is sufficient to cause the return of inflammatory pain within the hour. This phenomenon is so sensitive that even not following one's nutritional instinct, in the sense of not following one's instinctive attraction and eating randomly, is enough for inflammatory pain to return. The following example illustrates the point:

We have seen people in terminal phases of cancer who started eating instinctively when traditional medicine could not offer any more help. One particular case was a woman with breast cancer. Her tumor had developed to a point where it generated an open wound on her chest the size of a plate. At this stage of the disease, she could only survive by being constantly on morphine. Otherwise, her pain would have been unbearable. After only one week on Genefit, she was able to progressively reduce the use of morphine, and during the course of the second week, she was able to stop it completely. Every time she chose a food by will instead of interrogating her instinct, or every time she overate even slightly by pushing consumption a little too far after the unpleasant phase, her pain returned within the hour and lasted half a day to a day. Here, we are not talking about a little inflammatory pain, but pain no one could be expected to manage without appropriate medication. She ended up selecting foods blindfolded at every meal so as not to be influenced by her intellect.

Over time, inflammatory pain has actually become an amazingly precise criterion for us to define the limits of what can be considered a truly natural diet, and so check both the quality of food and the quality of one's practice. This is where the *pain = error* equation takes on vital importance. If you decide to eat according to the principles of Genefit Nutrition and you experience pain in any way, such as digestive pain, inflammatory pain, muscular pain, or any other discomfort, then there is, or has been, a mistake somewhere in your practice, in your food supply, or in the presence of either incoming or outgoing abnormal molecules in the bloodstream. Pain coming directly or indirectly from food doesn't exist under true instinctive eating conditions. Instead of taking a painkiller, as many people do, it is far more useful to discover the pain's origin in order to fix it. If you follow a Genefit Nutrition way of eating, use pain or even slight discomfort to help you become more precisely aware of your nutritional instinct and improve the quality of your food supply.

Another example of how precise the application of Genefit Nutrition must be in order to receive its full benefits is shown by what happens during viral diseases. Again, we have observed this result many times in many different people. Influenza is mostly a symptom-free experience for people on Genefit Nutrition when all the required conditions for instinctive eating are fulfilled, including strict food-supply-quality guidelines. During the course of viral disease, such as the flu, when one consumes even a small quantity of a food that doesn't fit in the unprocessed food specifications, such as steamed vegetables or even a spoon of honey that has been heated for comb extraction, the symptoms occur within a few hours, with the usual runny nose, headaches, and fever.

Inflammatory pain and the increase of symptoms during viral processes are two major criteria that helped us define what is natural unprocessed food and what is not. For food to be unprocessed, several conditions are required:

- No exposure to temperatures under 0°C/32°F at any time
- No exposure to temperatures over 40°C/104°F at any time
- No exposure to mechanical alteration (smashing, slicing, juicing, etc.)
- No exposure to irradiation
- No mixing or seasoning
- No overhybridized vegetal products such as wheat and corn
- No genetically modified food
- No selectively bred animals (beef, sheep, etc.) if use of animal products
- No meat from animals fed foods that do not match the present requirements
- No exposure to pesticides and commercial fertilizers
- No exposure to heated compost, if possible

The above quality requirements are not the result of some ideology. They have not been arbitrarily dictated out of an ideal of a pure diet. Each of these requirements is the result of four decades of experiments, trial and error, and observations. We have been able to determine the clear limits within which the nutritional instinct works, and how the body reacts when introducing food that has been processed, even in the slightest way, for people on Genefit Nutrition from several days to several decades. Similarly, we have observed how the body reacts under nonordinary circumstances, with the presence of pathological conditions such as viral processes or infectious diseases. Over time, it has become more and more clear that food processing alters the manner in which the body functions in the most unexpected and detrimental ways. The demarcation line between unprocessed and processed food is extremely sharp, and depending on what is on your daily table, you won't feel the same and you won't get the same results.

Experiments 3A and 3B demonstrate one of the major foundations Genefit Nutrition was built on. The more a food is processed, the more the change of taste or alliesthesial response gets blurry; it becomes literally nonexistent after a certain degree of processing. For example, small wild mangoes, as found on nonhybridized, ungrafted trees, have an absolute clear-cut alliesthesial response. If you eat them past your body's needs, the painful phase takes the form of a burning sensation in the mouth and throat, which can't be ignored. If you eat a Kent mango, or a Tommy Atkins, which are varieties that have been artificially hybridized and artificially selected to be easier to eat and sweeter, those mangoes will never burn your mouth. After a certain quantity has been eaten, they simply turn tasteless. One can easily overeat artificially selected mangos. If you add pieces of mango into a fruit salad, the change of taste disappears completely. When mangos are mixed with other fruits and sugar, the change of taste is gone, even if one eats large quantities. One can still find a slight alliesthesial response with a Kent mango by stopping when the flavor disappears, but there is clearly an open door to overeating.

Similarly, even slight increases in temperature may modify a food's molecular structure enough to make it impossible to evaluate it instinctively. For example, it is a common commercial practice to heat honey in order to remove it from the honeycomb and/or make it easier to pour into jars. Our taste-change mechanism will not function correctly with honey so treated. Unprocessed honey sooner or later produces an unpleasant taste to stop us from eating any more. Denatured honey does not. It can be eaten to excess, producing inflammatory tendencies, nausea, allergic reactions, and an abundance of other symptoms.

Inadvertent cooking may also denature other seemingly "natural" foods. There is practically no dried fruit of any sort on the commercial market today that has not at some stage of production been heated well above 104°F. In some cases, it is done to save time, in others to prevent the growth of fungus or mold. Drying in the sun also usually exceeds the 104°F mark. By treating the fruit with boiling water, drying it in the sun, or irradiating it, the producers unwittingly increase demand for their product, since it will fail to trigger a taste change, allowing far more to be eaten than is needed.

Nuts available in health food stores are always either frozen to kill insect eggs or dried at a high temperature to avoid mold. These nuts have no gustatory alliesthesia; the change of taste simply does not occur. The proof is that some raw food diets exclude them completely from the palette because people become addicted to them, eating abnormally large quantities. The consumption of those nuts brings back inflammatory pain and the usual symptoms of viral diseases in people who had avoided those problems thanks to Genefit Nutrition. Besides an immediate effect, health problems have been observed in the long run in people regularly eating processed nuts, due to a constant protein overload. Of course, truly unprocessed nuts are perfectly fine for the body. They are even necessary because they contain valuable nutrients. Excluding them completely from the palette is not a solution and can produce dietary imbalance over time. The only real solution to this problem is to find unheated, unfrozen nuts, so that the instinct can take over and regulate their intake.

Truly raw walnuts, for instance, have a thin skin around the flesh that tastes extremely bitter when the body doesn't need them. Sometimes people even spend a lot of time removing the skin so they can eat more of them without being bothered by the unpleasant taste. Of course, if you do this, it tricks your instinct. It is a form of processing. When walnuts are processed with heat, as is usually the case for those found in health food stores, the bitterness drastically drops, so people can eat them beyond the body's needs.

Few people are aware of all the treatment and processing techniques applied to "natural" foods, because with a traditional diet it isn't very important, since most food will be further processed in the kitchen. With Genefit Nutrition, it does matter. Hidden processing techniques are the traps you will have to avoid if you are planning to take on eating instinctively. Sometimes you cannot know if a food is processed because it does not always show. The external appearance may seem perfectly fine, but with Genefit Nutrition, you need to make sure the food is unaltered at a molecular level. When we think nutrition we often forget to think chemistry, but, in fact, nutrition is primarily chemistry. When soil transforms into a tree it is thanks to the miracle of chemistry. When a tree bears fruit it is also thanks to the miracle of chemistry. When our metabolism breaks the nutrients contained in a fruit down (catabolize) to an assimilable form, it is again thanks to the miracle of chemistry. And finally, when the body uses those building blocks to build muscles (anabolize) or to provide the chemicals necessary for the brain to work, it is thanks to the miracle of chemistry. All these steps are orchestrated by DNA, which is in itself also a result of complex chemistry. All this to say that when we think of nutrition, we should think of molecules and atoms, because in its most primary form, that's what it is. The slightest molecular alteration in a food can break the chain of chemical processing nature has intended. If we place so much importance on having a perfect food supply, it is not because we are somehow obsessed with the idea, but because experience has shown that, otherwise, the practice of Genefit Nutrition becomes imbalanced and even impossible.

In supermarkets and even in health food stores, the "traps" are numerous. The lack of awareness of the problems caused by processing did not hinder growers and producers from applying the most unexpected treatments and processing techniques. For example, fish such as swordfish are regularly frozen on the catch boat. Your local vendor may tell you his swordfish is fresh because he didn't freeze it, but in reality it was frozen before it came to the retail store and this is enough to create problems. Dates are almost always frozen to kill insects. Mangoes are always treated with hot water because of the very strict USDA requirements for impor-tation in the U.S. Corn has been genetically engineered and so produces abnormal proteins that do not match the body's genetic makeup with the result that the change of taste again does not occur. The same is true for the overselected avocado: Fuerte, Hass, etc., and the list goes on and on.

For those who plan to practice Genefit Nutrition over a long period of time, real detective work needs to be done to get the best possible food supply. With experience, you will get to know the most common pro-cessing techniques and learn how to avoid them. The most effective way to acquire unprocessed food is to go where food is produced or grown. Slowly build up a list of producers you can trust and you know are not using unwanted treatments. In buying from them, you will financially support those who really care about quality. They will be compensated for their hard work and hopefully motivated to continue it. This entire situation brought us to create The Purefood Network, a nonprofit organ-ization dedicated to providing Genefit Nutrition-friendly foods and sup-porting the growers and farmers who produce them. The profits from The Purefood Network are reinvested in land, which can then be assigned to farmers interested in producing Genefit Nutrition-quality foods. More information about The Purefood Network is available at the end of this book.

Foods in their natural state cannot poison a person with a trained nutritional instinct, but denatured mushrooms, on the other hand, can be deadly, since instinctive evaluation does not work. Many studies have been published on the types of mushrooms we can cook and still eat (with seasoning to make them gustarorily interesting) without harm. Here again intellectual intervention and knowledge is necessary not only to stay healthy but to stay alive.

With processed food, there is no safety net against imbalance because there is no dietary guidance. Once one has experienced the state of mind and body provided by Genefit Nutrition, one becomes aware that there is a huge loss of quality of life and health when one reintroduces a single processed food. With even slight exposure to processed food, the body doesn't work the same way, and the brain and nervous system don't work the way they are supposed to either. Over time, we have been able to define a specific *Genefit Nutritional state of reference* — a state one experiences when the food supply is a hundred percent correct, instinctive attraction to food is followed in a very precise manner, and instinctive stops are listened to perfectly. The psycho-psychological state induced by Genefit Nutrition is characterized by the following:

1. The digestion is always light and totally symptom free and profound satisfaction occurs without any pressure or sensation of volume in the stomach. It feels like radiant warmth extending from the stomach to the whole body, even if food is cold. It feels like radiant joy coming from the belly, producing a light state of euphoria.
2. Nearly symptom-free viral processes: When the body has been thoroughly cleansed, viral processes tend to occur without the usual symptoms. The body develops the capacity to control or even use these so-called "diseases" for its own benefit without any harm or discomfort.
3. The absence of inflammatory pain regardless of the severity of the condition expected to trigger it under traditional eating conditions.
4. An outstanding quietness and clarity of mind: the absence of abnormal molecules circulating in the brain permits a general relaxation of the nervous system, which is remarkably higher than one can experience under traditional eating conditions. Along with an improved control over the mind stream, you will notice the absence of chaotic dreams and nightmares.

With Genefit Nutrition, the presence of these four criteria provides confirmation of a completely correct food supply. Now, let us suppose you have been on Genefit Nutrition for at least a few months, and everything has been going well. You feel great until suddenly, you lose one or more of the criteria above. In order to fix the problem, you should first question your food supply to see if there might be a food that goes outside the limits of the definition of unprocessed food. If no such food is found, the next step is to determine if you find yourself in the middle of a useful detox wave, which can temporarily cause a loss of life quality. The next step is to question your practice of Genefit Nutrition. You might have overlooked an alliesthesial response, or you might not have taken enough time to use your senses carefully. If neither of these explanations applies, the fourth recommended step is to question Genefit

Nutrition itself. There are things we might not have seen despite decades of research and observation. Most of the time, you won't have to go much further than the first step: checking the food supply quality. Once you have eliminated the problem food from your palette, the desired state of your body will soon return. People who skip the first three steps of this process may easily be misled to believe that Genefit Nutrition doesn't work.

The Genefit Nutritional experiment is unique. It goes against the current — the general tendency — and as a result, a considerable effort will be needed to stay away from food processing. If your food palette is completely unprocessed, and if you pay careful attention to your nutritional instinct, you will be pleasantly surprised at how your body and nervous system work. Wild animals that don't have access to human garbage and man-made food have an advantage. They never have to worry about their food supply; nature automatically provides the right one. Our ancestors who started food processing probably had no idea of what they got us into. Processing has conquered both the world and our stomachs.

The phenomena involved with Genefit Nutrition are so subtle that tiny amounts of processed food can limit them, or in some cases eliminate them altogether. Since humans started processing their food, there are only few a people who have experienced how it feels to live exclusively on unprocessed foods. As a result, nobody has ever before been able to define the specific state one enters when the body returns to its original way of functioning.

What is commonly considered standard by the medical profession is inaccurate because of the metabolic distortions processing techniques bring along. The effects processed foods have on the body are today still largely underestimated. On the other hand, the effects one experiences with Genefit Nutrition are, nonetheless, reproducible at any time by anybody who chooses to apply it accurately.

THE PROS AND CONS OF MEAT

What food is really "natural" for us as a species? Are we "naturally" (i.e., genetically) carnivorous, omnivorous, fructivorous, or something else?

There are numerous schools of thought on this subject, some of them of a religious nature, others philosophical, still others founded on scientific enquiry. There is generally little agreement among them. Some people currently object to eating meat. It has been argued on philosophical grounds that we should not eat meat because it is immoral to slaughter animals but this issue is closer to theology than nutrition. In addition, it would be disrespectful to argue with people who exclude meat for moral reasons. Everyone must choose for himself and be consistent with his beliefs.

On other grounds, the argument has been advanced that humans are not meant to eat meat because we lack the incisors and claws of carnivores such as tigers and minks. Paradoxically, some rodents, equipped with both claws and incisors, are predominantly vegetarian rather than carnivorous, and carnivores may also eat vegetable foods on occasion. In fact, many animals are actually more omnivorous than is suggested by the either-or categories of classical zoology. A cow getting proteins from insects and snails unavoidably mixed with grass, and a lion eating predigested grass from the guts of an antelope, support this claim.

From an evolutionary point of view, primate and hominid meat eating is not a recent behavior. Chimpanzees are known to occasionally hunt small monkeys or rodents for their meat and have probably done so for a long time.

Many people have discovered, in fact, that their health improved when they avoided meat. What few of them ever noticed, however, is that their health improved when they stopped eating *cooked* meat. Meat in its native state is a different matter. It is regularly seen that under instinctive eating conditions healthy infants and children, as well as adults, are spontaneously attracted to the smells and tastes of various meats. But, they consume significantly less meat than the majority of the population living on cooked foods. So the inference can be made that we are relatively noncarnivorous, but only relatively so. Vegetarians and vegans may choose to practice Genefit Nutrition without recourse to meat. One can obtain a great deal of protein from nuts, legumes, and other plant sources. But remember, plant proteins and seed foods are not whole-animal foods, and cannot entirely substitute for them.

From experience, we have seen that under instinctive eating conditions, raw meat can bring the best and the worst. The best, because there have been the most astonishing recoveries with consumption of raw meat. Leukemia and other forms of cancer can sometimes improve quickly when large quantities of raw meat are temporarily eaten within instinctive evaluation. Apparently, meat sometimes supplies either healing potentials or detox opportunities that may help the body rid itself of symptoms from those pathologies. And precisely for that reason, we never exclude it completely from the Genefit Nutritional food palette. Excluding meat up front would take away the opportunity the body might need to improve serious conditions. On the other hand, we have also observed cases of fast-growing tumors in people who ate excessively large quantities of raw meat over several years. Those quantities were not regulated by the nutritional instinct. How did this happen?

Meat is a very powerful food, and at the same time, a very sensitive one. It is a sensitive food because it doesn't take much to get meat outside our definition of unprocessed food. For a better understanding of this phenomenon, we need to keep in mind that any organism "is" what it eats. Feed a pig garbage and his meat will have a garbage aftertaste. Crayfish raised in muck will taste of muck.

The dangers of man-made toxins such as mercury in fish or pesticides on fruit are widely recognized. The dangers of man-made toxins in the form of industrial food for pigs or chickens, oats and heated hay for horses, wheat and supplements for cattle are too often not taken into consideration. Some of those foods may be "natural" foods in that they are products of nature (although probably denatured by artificial selection), but unless they were part of the eater's native alimentary spectrum, they are unnatural for it, and will produce unnatural effects in it, and subsequently, in whatever feeds upon it.

From this perspective, is wheat a natural food for cattle? Cattle are fed grains in order to artificially put weight on them. If someone is selling a product by the pound, the more pounds he sells the more money he makes. In our society, this is not only allowed but encouraged. We have come to value *more*, and for most of us, bigger has become better. Mother is proud that her baby is big. The gardener is proud of his big tomatoes. We prefer not to raise small children, small fruit, or small cattle. So we feed our children, our beasts, and fertilize our produce with whatever will increase their volume and weight. Cows do not get fat on grass, but on grains, or in more general terms, on foods to which their biochemistry is not genetically adapted. This observation applies to any animal, and it certainly applies to humans. Humans get fat on bread, cooked sugars, cooked potatoes, milk, cheese, and most other denatured food their bodies can only partially digest, but have learned to tolerate.

When an animal eats processed food or food that doesn't match its genetic makeup, abnormal molecules contained in that food enter its body. Abnormal molecules from denatured food can only be partially used, and partially eliminated, because they are alien to the body's built-in biochemical programming. What happens to whatever has not been metabolized, not used, and not discarded? It remains. And over time, more and more of these chemicals are stored in the animal's cellular tissues, the ones we may end up eating.

Most domesticated animals get a daily load of abnormal molecules along with their feed ration. Those abnormal molecules alter the taste of their meat, so the nutritional instinct is misled, opening the way to overeating. For meat to be completely appropriate for Genefit Nutritional consumption, it must come from animals that have not been eating any food that goes outside the definition of unprocessed food for two complete generations. Otherwise, the nutritional instinct responds poorly to it. When raw meat is repeatedly consumed outside the body's needs, the intake exceeds the body's digestive capacity, and entire strings of foreign proteins enter the bloodstream and the lymph system. Those foreign proteins have the "building shape" of the animal they come from, and are therefore foreign to the human body. They can, when several conditions are reunited, create random mutations when the human body's cells duplicate, and boost the production of cancer cells. Ironically, the proteins coming from mammals are the most dangerous ones, because they are the closest to our own proteins, so the immune system might not always recognize them as foreign and might allow them to accumulate freely in the body.

The only solution to this problem is the nutritional instinct, with the right quantity of meat, consumed at the right time. But, for the nutritional instinct to work, meat must be absolutely free from abnormal molecules coming from artificial feeding. Furthermore, and this will reduce our choice in meats, selectively bred animals like sheep, beef, and pork have a tendency to produce a poor gustatory alliesthesia, which enables overeating in the same way hybridized fruits do. The difference with fruits is that carbohydrates are far less dangerous than animal proteins when overeaten.

Excluding meat from the palette is not the solution since some people obviously need it. But, if meat is introduced in the palette, it should be done with wild game that has not undergone artificial feeding. Strictly unfed wild game is the guarantee against overeating and health problems. With this type of meat, the instinctive stop is completely accurate, and we have never observed a problem with it, even over time. Unfed wild game has a painful phase (the taste turns really bad when the body doesn't need it). On the other hand, selectively bred meat does not. It is also important to note that with the meat of wild game, there are no signs of inflammatory pain after consumption, which strongly suggests that meat in its truly original state is natural for the human body. Another common problem we have encountered with meat, and especially wild game, is freezing. Meat is almost always frozen in slaughterhouses. So care must be taken when procuring meat for consumption since the nutritional instinct also fails with frozen meat.

For the above reasons, we have seen people eat large quantities of meat even if their body didn't need it, and this is exactly when problems are likely to occur, because the accumulation of undigested proteins reaches a certain level especially after years of overeating. Raw meat can be the most wonderful therapeutic food, but it is also the most dangerous one of all when eaten outside the body's needs. Except for very specific cases, and then only temporarily, meat is a very small part of the food palette of Genefit Nutrition. Many vitamins and other nutrients contained in meat can be obtained in many other foods, such as seafood, for instance. It is perfectly safe to eat meat only occasionally, if the food palette contains a sufficiently diverse choice of other animal products.

For those interested in a limited cleanse of twenty-one days or so, we recommend that meat be omitted, since it is so difficult to get the proper quality. Unless you really feel the need to integrate meat into the program, it is better to concentrate on other foods your body might need. You won't suffer from any deficiency because of the absence of meat if you practice Genefit Nutrition for just a few weeks. Most people have a tendency to eat far too much meat while on a traditional diet. Once on Genefit Nutrition, it is good to give your body a rest and a chance to adjust possible overloads.

For those who plan to apply Genefit Nutrition for a longer period of time, we would suggest that you not exclude unprocessed meat up front, even if the idea of eating raw meat doesn't appeal to you. A philosophical or psychological impediment might deprive you of nutrients you need. If during your practice, you have the opportunity to acquire real unprocessed meat that matches our quality guidelines, at least smell it. Give your nutritional instinct a chance to tell you whether you need it or not. If there is no instinctive attraction, that is, if it doesn't smell good, don't eat it. But if it does smell good, at least consider trying it.

Remember that with Genefit Nutrition, there is no coercion; eat only what tastes good. Many people start on Genefit Nutrition with no intention whatsoever of eating meat, and that is perfectly fine. They can do well without meat for several years on this diet. Then, at some point, they may encounter truly natural meat and will eat a large quantity because it smelled extremely good. After this experience, they might not eat meat for another six months. But, if you are thinking of eating meat regularly, make sure you get the right quality. Otherwise, you will be defeating the purpose of the program. It is better not to eat meat at all than to compromise on the quality.

NONHUMAN FOOD

Any food that could not have been consumed by human beings a million years ago (before we planted seeds or invented ropes for cattle and pots) cannot truly be food for us now. There are two major types of nonhuman foods that we mistakenly consume with detrimental effects: dairy products and grains.

1. Dairy Products

Our distant forebears didn't drink the milk of animals. Before cows were domesticated, a wild cow would hardly have stood still long enough to

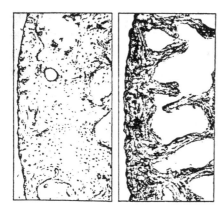

FIGURE 6. Comparison between bone structure of Neanderthals and modern humans.

be milked. Even assuming our ancestors were interested in doing it, and someone had figured out how, they would have needed a vessel to hold the milk. No such item had been invented. We might imagine a group of distant prehistoric men surrounding a wild cow, and taking turns suckling her teats, but it seems unlikely. If we look around us in nature, we find no cases of one species of mammal ingesting the milk of another. We do not see squirrels suckling goats or weasels suckling foxes. Nor do we find an adult member of a species ingesting milk at all, only the offspring. From this we can infer that even same-species milk is unnatural for adults.

Our culture holds that cow's milk is a "natural" food, and that babies and children need calcium from it in order to grow strong bones and teeth. But the fossil record tells us that our prehistoric ancestors had strong bones and teeth without cow's milk. Their bones were less brittle than ours, and fractured less readily.

Let's look at a microscopically polarized bone cross-section of a Neanderthal man's finger joint:

As compared with modern man, the distribution of calcium is entirely different. In the first case, bone structure is dense and haphazard, which makes for flexibility and resilience, whereas in modern man, calcium has precipitated so much that bone structure has expanded, making the bone hard and brittle.

Note: Wild animals and Neanderthal man share the same bone structure, since neither feeds on milk of another species.

If early humans had truly needed nonhuman milk to survive, they would not have survived. Even unprocessed dairy products, such as raw milk, do not produce a change of taste. Human's exposure to cow's milk is only ten thousand years old, which is extremely short in terms of evolutionary history.

Experience has shown us that dairy products create health problems when introduced into an instinctive diet. For example, infections never happen among people on Genefit Nutrition, even if the wounds are not cleaned. (For the sake of science, people who first experimented with the principles of eating instinctively have even put dirt into existing accidental cuts. It was impossible to create an infection.) But, infections have been observed in people using dairy products along with Genefit Nutrition. When dairy products are part of the food palette, the body does not have the same immunological resistance. In addition, dairy products make it impossible to reach the typical Genefit Nutritional state of reference.

The most amusing example confirming a nonadaptation to dairy products is . . . smelly feet. People dislike unpleasant body odors, because they are not natural. Pigs in captivity smell terrible, in comparison to wild boars. As you probably have guessed, the difference lies in the food they eat and the conditions they live in. Abnormal body odors are the result of the ejection of abnormal molecules. Experience always confirms this view: children who eat instinctively from birth do not have unpleasant body odors, even if they do not bathe every day.

The ejection of previously accumulated abnormal molecules is the body's emergency response to a dietary situation that can produce serious health problems. Abnormal body odors are an early sign that the body has trouble dealing with the molecules and toxins. The body attempts to get rid of these impurities through any means available, mainly through the intestine and perspiration, which are the biggest, most accessible, detoxification paths.

The following is the example of Veronique, who had been on Genefit Nutrition for many years. After such an amount of time, her body had barely any odor, and then only very occasionally, during detoxification waves. Once, Veronique went to a family meeting for a few days and attended endless lunches and dinners, which were of course, cooked.

Veronique ate, among other things, a minor quantity of cheese. The following night, her perspiration and feet started to smell like the cheese she had eaten. She had not experienced this type of body odor for years, but it returned after only *one* episode of cheese consumption. It took a few days back on Genefit Nutrition for the smell to disappear completely and permanently. In the case of Veronique, the link between smelly feet and the consumption of dairy products is as clear as can be. This example is of importance, primarily because it logically leads us to the following two conclusions:

1. First, the molecules contained in cheese are unwanted by the body, otherwise it wouldn't make such an effort to get rid of them. One never smells like an orange after consuming oranges, especially if they were instinctively evaluated. The difference between these two foods lies in the body's genetic adaptation to them. The body is genetically adapted to the molecules of the orange because the orange or the "orange's ancestors" have always been around during our evolutionary history. Exposure to dairy products has occurred over too short a time for our bodies to adapt. The body struggles with the molecules of cheese and does everything it can to expel them, even through extraordinary pathways. The rapidness of the reaction of the body indicates a state of emergency. Experience shows those molecules are dangerous to the human body. Again, they are dangerous only because the body is genetically not adapted to them.

2. The second conclusion is that the cheese molecules carry the same odor on their way out as they had on their way in. There has not been any molecular transformation in between. If they had been broken down by digestion, as should have been the case, they would smell differently or have no odor at all. This observation demonstrates that those molecules skipped the process of digestion and entered the body undigested. Undigested molecules coming from another species wandering around in the organism are highly dangerous; they can easily provoke mutations leading to cancer, autoimmune diseases, and many other severe problems. A foreign protein is only able to enter the body unaltered and create harm if the body does not have the appropriate enzymes to digest it, which also means that the body is not genetically adapted to that specific protein.

This is how smelly feet indicate the harmfulness of dairy products and so we have chosen to exclude dairy products completely from our daily palette. There is just too much evidence against them, both from our own experience and from work done by other researchers and practitioners.

2. *Grains and Cereals*

Our ancient predecessors didn't eat rice or wheat. They might have stumbled onto a growth of wild rice and explored the taste of its grains. They might even have liked it. Human beings today do not generally care for, or manage to eat, uncooked rice, although many birds and rodents enjoy it. Furthermore, rice would have been scarce. It was only eight to ten thousand years ago that humans began to cultivate cereals. Over the millions of years preceding agriculture, it seems unlikely that rice would have been plentiful enough to provide much food. In fact, it seems improbable that any cereal would have been on our ancestral menu. Wild wheat, barleycorn, or oats might have been of occasional passing interest. But without methods of cultivating them in quantity, they could have provided only a very small part of evolving humankind's nutrition. Even assuming an abundance of one or another of these grains, the problem of threshing them a handful at a time would not have made them very practical or popular.

Sprouted garbanzo beans, lentils, or other grains might occasionally be on the Genefit Nutrition menu, but wheat, corn, and soy specifically, have been excluded from the palette because of the overhybridization, artificial selection, and genetic engineering they have undergone.

> The foods we eat are usually divided into four basic groups: meat and fish, vegetables and fruit, milk and milk products, and breads and cereals. Two or more daily servings from each are now considered necessary for a balanced diet, but adults living before the development of agriculture and animal husbandry got all their nutrients from the first two food groups: they apparently consumed cereal grains rarely if at all, and they had no dairy foods whatsoever (S.B. Eaton and M. Kowner, *Paleolithic Nutrition* [*The New England Journal of Medicine*, Jan., 1985]).

SEVEN

The Nose Knows

EXPERIMENT 4

This experiment works best in the morning on an empty stomach.

Buy a choice of five or six of the fruits you like most (preferably organic). Try to choose, by intuition or with your mind, the specific fruit that might most closely fit your body's needs. But don't eat it. Simply remember your choice.

Now start using your sense of smell. Put all the fruit in a row in front of you and start smelling one after another. Take your time. It might take a while for your instinct to become fully active. Ten to fifteen minutes is a reasonable time to spend. You will notice changes in the perception of the odors. A fruit that can smell good at first can begin to smell bad after some time. Pay attention to these changes. Look only for the pleasantness of the smell and not the intensity. If you find an unpleasant component in the smell of a given fruit, eliminate that option right away and put it aside. As soon as the odor of a fruit turns bad or unpleasant after a second or third smelling attempt, omit that fruit. If you don't perceive an odor, scratch the skin of the fruit. Proceed with the same process until only one fruit is left. This is the fruit chosen by your instinct.

The fruit you choose first with your mind rarely matches the one your instinct chose. Your instinct chooses in order to fit your body's needs. Your intellect chooses from criteria like memories, convenience, and habits. The experiment helps us to distinguish between instinct and intelligence.

This experiment works better if you blindfold yourself and ask someone to help you smell. It is much easier to focus on the instinct and to follow it without visual stimulation.

CHEMOTAXIS IS THE SCIENTIFIC TERM for the capacity of bacteria to chemically analyze "food particles" in the vicinity. Chemotaxis helps a bacterium determine whether a given food particle will be beneficial or harmful before being "swallowed" through a process called phagocytosis or endocytosis.

The need to eat the right food at the right time has been an issue for living organisms since life first appeared on Earth. Even a life form as simple as a bacterium needs the right guidance when it comes to its diet. Otherwise, survival becomes compromised.

Bacteria and other single-cell organisms have an extremely high mutation rate. The shorter the lifespan of an organism, the higher the chances of mutations over a given period of time. For example, a new human generation occurs every twenty-five years or so. Within those twenty-five years, if bacteria have an average life span of about seven days, they will give birth to 1,300 new generations. This means that the rate of genetic adaptability is 1,300 times higher in bacteria than it is for human beings, or we could also say bacteria adapt to their environment at least 1,300 times faster than human beings.

Bacteria and single-cell animals using chemotaxis or similar tools ruled the world for about a billion years before the appearance of multicellular animals, such as plankton, algae, and jellyfish. At a rate of a new generation every seven days, we would obtain something like fifty-two billion generations between the first cells equipped with chemotaxis and the appearance of more complex multicellular animals. Over time, each generation faced all kinds of new dietary problems, and they had to solve them in order to stay alive. Consequently, bacteria with chemotaxis not working efficiently perished. Only the cells responding positively to new situations reproduced. And, billions of generations later, we obtain only cells where the chemotactic function works at its best, regardless of the complexity of the situation encountered. The resulting accumulated experience is enormous. Considering the evolutionary history of single-cell organisms alone, we can already see that the nutritional fine-tuning achieved by the nutritional instinct is extraordinary. Since we retain parts of the DNA of those early bacteria in our own DNA, we have, to a certain extent, inherited the benefits of their experience.

Roughly one billion years ago, the first multicellular animals formed from single-cell organisms. And again, they faced the same nutritional problem: eat the right food at the right time, in the right quantity. Much later, animals such as reptiles or mammals developed specialized cells, known as gustatory and olfactory receptors, connected to corresponding brain centers to chemically analyze food. From bacteria to apes, the nutritional instinct evolved over numerous generations across numerous species to become a tool of extraordinary complexity, expressing itself through the senses of taste and smell. It is true that whether we consider bacteria or apes, the problem of achieving dietary balance always stays the same.

Chemotaxis gives us an idea of how old the nutritional instinct is. Chemotaxis, and what later became a complex alimentary sensory system, has constantly been improving over the three billion years of life evolution. The nutritional instinct is as old as life itself, because the problem of finding the right food and eating it in the right quantity has been there since the beginning.

Humans are the only animals in evolutionary history that tried to solve the dietary problem with their minds. Although analytic capacities present many advantages, which certainly have helped us to survive and conquer the planet, can our neocortex really compete with three billion years of experience? Let's not forget that conceptual intelligence is, at most, two million years old. Animals other than humans never came to use intelligence, because they had the perfect tool available right in the middle of their faces: the nose. Chimpanzees never eat anything without smelling it first. The same is true of other mammals, such as dogs, rodents, etc.

The sense of smell is a biological wonder and its accuracy is truly amazing. Within our nasal passages, the human olfactory epithelium contains some ten million cells that are constantly in touch with the air. The sensation of smell is the result of specific airborne molecules striking specialized sensor cells in the nose, which then react by sending electrical signals to the brain, where the sensation of smell actually happens. For animals, smelling is a sensory question mark, and when a food is smelled, it becomes a dietetic question: "Does my body need this food or not?" For every such dietary question, there is an answer, and the answer lies in the pleasantness of smell. It really is as simple as that. The pleasantness of smell tells whether or not a given food is beneficial to the body. If animals in nature are to survive, needed foods must smell good as long as they are needed, and unneeded or poisonous foods must smell unattractive. It would also be imperative that odors associated with danger and sexuality trigger the proper reactions for a species to thrive. But there would be no reason for mechanisms to evolve with respect to smells that were irrelevant to survival.

An interesting experiment was carried out by a physiology research group in Lyon, France, to explore how odors varied before and after eating. Two groups of volunteers were first asked to rate the pleasantness/ unpleasantness of ten different substances on a scale of -2 (very unattractive) to 0 (neutral) to +2 (very attractive). Three groups of test items were used: 1) food odors: meat, fish, and honey; 2) odors from nonfoods frequently associated with foods: tobacco, wine, and coffee; and 3) nonfood odors: lavender, sodium hypochlorite, and India ink.

After rating the odors, one group had a meal of bread, butter, ham, french-fries, concentrated sweet milk, and an orange. The control group simply didn't eat. After the meal, both groups were asked to smell and rate each sample seven times at twenty-minute intervals.

The before and after ratings of the food odors were markedly different. Before eating, the food odors were almost universally attractive to both groups. Presumably, some differences in ratings were a result of personal preferences or individual criteria for scoring. But however attractive a food odor may have been before the meal, its rating after the meal was significantly lower, while the control group, the ones who hadn't eaten, continued to find them attractive.

However, the meal, or lack of it, had no significant effect on the ratings of nonfood odors. Tobacco, coffee, wine, lavender, sodium hypochlorite, and ink smelled just as pleasant or unpleasant to the eaters after the meal as they had before, and also did not vary for the control group. Researchers concluded that we possess an alliesthesial mechanism that makes the smell of food relatively attractive when we feel hungry and unattractive when we don't. There is one necessary inference the researchers did not explicitly draw from the results of the experiment, possibly because it seemed obvious: the attractiveness or repulsiveness we experience when smelling a food directly depends on our body's biochemical state. We will not be attracted to a smell when our biochemistry isn't open to it.

You will discover, after eating by instinct for a time, that smells and tastes become clearer than ever before, and a clear-cut alliesthesial response with unprocessed foods will become as spontaneous and natu-

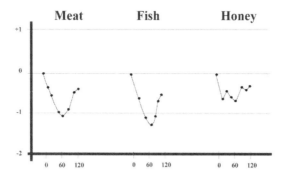

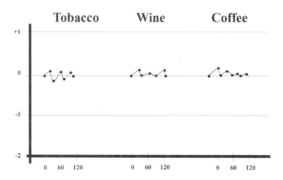

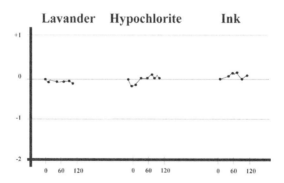

FIGURE 7. Duclaux, Feisthauer & Cabanac, "Effects of Eating a Meal on the Pleasantness of Food and Non-food Odors in Man," *Physiology and Behavior*, Vol. 10, 1973.

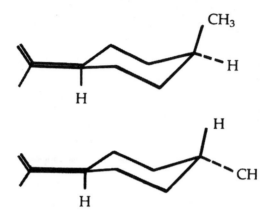

FIGURE 8. Stereochemical comparison.

ral as experiencing hot and cold. In fact, you will learn to recognize when a supposedly original food is not in its original state, because its taste doesn't change.

It has been assumed that we humans have lost our nutritional instinct. Four decades of experimentation indicates otherwise. If we are attracted to a food when we don't need it, then something must have gone wrong with our internal control and sensing systems. If we are not attracted to a food when we do need it, something must also be wrong. And it is easy to see what it is: millions of years of evolutionary development did not pre-pare our bodies or our built-in alimentary sensing systems (our instinct) to cope with denatured foods. Any particular smell or taste we experi-ence depends on both the structure of the incoming molecules and the biochemical state of the body. Even a slight change in structure, which does not affect the molecule's composition (i.e., its chemical formula), may dramatically alter its interactions with its surroundings. Both mole-cules pictured on page 93 have the same number of radicals, containing the same atoms, but they are placed differently. The trans-p-Menth-8-ene on the top smells like oranges. The cis-p-Menth-8-ene on the bottom smells like crude oil. Unless analyzed by stereochemical methods or our noses, they are *chemically* the same.

The new smell from a stew made from the ingredients mentioned above results from molecules with a new structure reaching receptor cells in the nose. No single ingredient smelled that way at the outset, nor did the original uncooked collection of them. The stew's new taste is unlike the taste of any single ingredient within it, due to molecules with new structures coming into contact with receptor cells on the tongue. The novel odor and taste of any cooked food is the product of molecular structures not found in nature. For the most part, we find them fascinating. Otherwise, what would have been the point of concocting them in the first place?

A raw potato doesn't smell the same as a cooked one, because of differences in the molecular structure of the aromatic molecules. Our sense of smell has developed in contact with aromatic molecules coming from a natural unprocessed context. Olfactory information from natural molecules is the language the brain centers that are part of the nutritional instinct understand. Olfactory information from processed food is like an incomprehensible foreign language. Although it may sound fascinating there is just no way it can be decoded correctly. Olfactory cells and hypothalamic brain centers processing the information are built from blueprints coming from our genes, as is the case with any other organ in the body. Many genetic changes would be necessary for the nutritional instinct to understand a new molecular "language." As empirical evidence confirms, the nutritional instinct has not yet been able to adjust completely to new aromatic molecules.

Because of the advent of processed food, we can no longer rely on our nutritional instinct to guide us safely. Similarly, when our ancestors started processing food, the nutritional instinct suddenly ceased to give them appropriate information. It is not such a far stretch to imagine that they might have experienced symptoms such as a poor digestion after meals of processed food. After relying on their perfectly well-functioning instinct for dietary guidance for many generations, suddenly, with processed food, the more they followed the pleasantness of smell and taste, the sicker they got. The accumulation of bad experiences resulted in the loss of confidence in the nutritional instinct itself. Our ancestors progressively came to the conclusion that blindly following their senses of taste and smell — their nutritional instinct — leads to trouble, simply because recipes always smell and taste good, even though they cause digestive difficulties and other health issues. In fact, the nutritional instinct was still functioning properly; instead it was the change of food environment that was responsible for all kinds of symptoms. Since we are talking about events that took place some hundred thousand years ago, the first humans may have been unable to clearly analyze the relationship between cause and effect. Slowly over time, the idea that we have lost our nutritional instinct and, instead, need our intellect to regulate our diet became more and more integrated in our cultural belief system. This idea is right to a certain extent, because when food is processed, the intellect is the only mechanism left to somehow resolve dietary issues. With unprocessed food, we don't need the intellect, because the nutritional instinct has the right conditions in which to work. On an individual level, time and repetitive positive observations are needed to rebuild trust in our nutritional instinct. If you try Genefit Nutrition, slowly you will increase the awareness that listening to your own nutritional instinct is the shortest path to well being.

In our modern culture, the sense of smell is neglected and underdeveloped, because we have lost sight of its main purpose, which is to help us find the food that will make us healthy. Several studies conducted in the 1980s were intended to investigate the involvement of the senses of smell and taste in a human nutritional instinct. They failed, because the distinction between unprocessed and processed food was not made. Researchers were expecting gustatory and olfactory alliesthesia from processed food. Since those phenomena weren't observed, it was concluded that we couldn't rely on them to regulate our diet. Those studies concentrated mainly on sweet and salty tastes and tried to compare their pleasantness before and after consumption of a sweet or salty food. Slight differences have been found, which are probably signals from the nutritional instinct that managed to pass trough the obstruction shield produced by food processing. Those signals are not accurate enough to regulate one's diet effectively, however, and we do not advocate using them. They are a degenerated form of the very precise and complex alliesthesia one can experience with unprocessed food.

In the right context, the sense of smell gives us a real-time report of the body's needs without having to taste every food. Olfactory attraction is the signal that attracts us to the best food currently available, the one that best matches our bodies' need. Animals have the same experience.

Chimpanzees looking for food in the rainforest sometimes smell a fruit tree before they even see it. Fruit trees are hard to recognize by sight among the luxurious vegetation characteristic of tropical forests. Fallen fruits and the leaves of trees are strongly odiferous because of the rainforest's warmth and humidity.

In order to easily understand how our sense of smell works, we need to place it in the context in which it evolved. To do this, imagine yourself walking in the rainforest with hundreds of incredible smells surrounding you. Some are more appealing than others. Your sense of smell will constantly adjust to the best possible food within smelling distance. The smell of this particular food will become predominant over all others, since it is the one that matters most to your body. If you continue your walk, and find yourself in a place where a better matching food is present, the smell of the new food will become predominant over the previous one. The smell of the previous food may even become unpleasant, or simply yield to the new one. This is how olfactory attraction can change within a few seconds. The odors of unprocessed foods can change like day and night. The flowery rich smell of cauliflower can become comparable to the terrible smell of dog feces, depending on the body's attractions or aversions. The change sometimes occurs instantly if the body finds a food that fits its needs better.

Unfortunately, since most of you will probably practice Genefit Nutrition at home and not in the rainforest, you will have to hold food right below your nose in order to focus carefully on your instinct. If you have never used your nutritional instinct before, it will be rusty and need some time and training. In the meantime, it will be difficult to smell foods from a distance. The pleasantness of smell, which is the positive signal of the body's needs, is not to be confused with the intensity of the smell. For example, a guava smells strong, independent of the body's needs. It is important to look for pleasant or unpleasant components of the guava's smell in order to decide whether to eat it. In the beginning, most people experience some difficulty in trying to distinguish between the two.

All complex instincts have what is called a sensitive period which is the period of brain development when the instinct expresses itself for the first time. Sensitive periods allow an instinct to adjust to the environment to a certain extent. It gives them the last touch they need to be completely in sync with the surroundings and become fully operational. The nutritional instinct also goes through such a sensitive period when it comes in contact with solid food for the first time in early childhood. The first retrieved information when this happens serves as a reference and calibrates the interpretation of the sensations of smell and taste in our brain. For most of us, the first solid food we came in contact with was cooked or processed, so the reference is not accurate. A conversion period is needed to integrate the innate tastes and smells of unprocessed food.

Just as repletion and the sense of taste work as a team, the sense of smell works with salivation. When the body wants a food, a salivation reflex accompanies the pleasantness of smell. Salivation is the first step of digestion, and when salivation occurs while smelling a food, it is a sign that the digestive system is ready to digest it. You have to be careful with this signal, because salivation can be induced by the mind. You might think of your favorite recipe, and the memory of its taste could trigger salivation, even if your body has no need for it. The salivation induced by memory is not a reflex. The salivation reflex we are referring to is not controlled by the conscious mind.

Sometimes the body might have a metabolic need for a particular food, but is, for various reasons, presently unable to digest it properly. In this case, there will be pleasantness of smell without the salivation reflex. When this happens it is recommended to test this specific food again during your next meals until the digestive system say yes to it. First, the pleasantness of smell is the indicator of metabolic needs, and second, the salivation reflex is the digestive green light for consumption.

Imagine yourself at an intersection with two traffic lights. As long as one is red, you are not supposed to move forward. With your nutritional instinct, wait until both lights turn green, pleasantness of smell and salivation reflex, before you start eating a particular food. So, remember, always scratch and sniff before eating; there is no better guarantee for a healthy life.

EIGHT

The Question that Drives Us

Repeat Experiment 4, day after day. You will notice that most of
the time your instinct will choose a different fruit from one day
to another. Your body's needs are changing from day to day. The
nutritional instinct is matching these needs as closely as possible,
within the given parameters.

SOME PEOPLE SAY they don't like one food or another, and won't
even try them. It seems perfectly reasonable. Why should someone force
himself to eat something he knows he doesn't like, or even taste something he's sure he won't like? Let's explore this question in greater detail:
Imagine a person named John. At some point during John's early childhood, in 1971 let us say, he was offered a tomato that he tasted and didn't
like. We'll call it Tomato 1. It was a raw tomato, unseasoned, in its original state. His biochemistry caused him to dislike it because he didn't
need it. However, his mother might have insisted he eat it, on the theory
that tomatoes are healthy foods, always and everywhere good for you.
Subjected often enough to this way of thinking, John might even come
to the conclusion that only bad-tasting foods were good for him, adopting as an unconscious nutritional credo: the worse it tastes, the better it
is. (This principle may even partially motivate widespread practices such
as wheat grass juicing.) Tomato 1 in Figure 9 (page 98) represents this
evil-tasting tomato that day in 1971.

In 2001 let us say, John may visit a friend's backyard garden where he
is offered a tomato: Tomato 2, which is also represented in Figure 9. John
is ready to eat everything else, but he will not touch the tomato. If you
ask him why, his reply will be, "Because I don't like tomatoes." "But you
haven't even tried it!" you might say, and John would answer, "I never

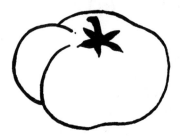 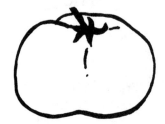

FIGURE 9. Tomato 1 and tomato 2.

liked them!" From his first bad experience with a tomato — just one may have been enough — John created a generalization about them. Tomato 1 and Tomato 2 look alike, their size, color, and shape are almost the same. So John assumes they must taste the same. He is unaware that the flavors of unprocessed foods are continually changing, unlike cooked foods. Furthermore, and here lies an insidious trap, Tomato 1 and Tomato 2 carry the same name. The very same label "Tomato" applies to both experiences, even though they may be separated by thirty years. But in John's mind, it seems perfectly rational to avoid anything that carries that name, because logically, for him, they are the same.

For those of us who find ourselves trapped like John, it might be rewarding, at least occasionally, to smell and taste a food we may not previously have liked, before we declare it *non grata*. In an unprocessed food environment, there is no way to tell from its name how something will taste at a given moment. With processed food, on the other hand, eating pleasure and pleasantness of taste are predictable. If someone orders a pizza, he or she can be sure that this pizza will provide eating pleasure, especially if he or she orders the same brand every time. The same happens with our favorite cookies, candies, even our favorite recipes. Once we have tasted a recipe, the next time we can foresee its taste and the level of eating pleasure it will provide. We consciously want to have eating pleasure, and we know that we will get it. The reverse is also true. If we have ordered a menu item that didn't taste good at one time, we won't order it a second time, because we know that it will taste the same. This phenomenon has much deeper consequences than one might think.

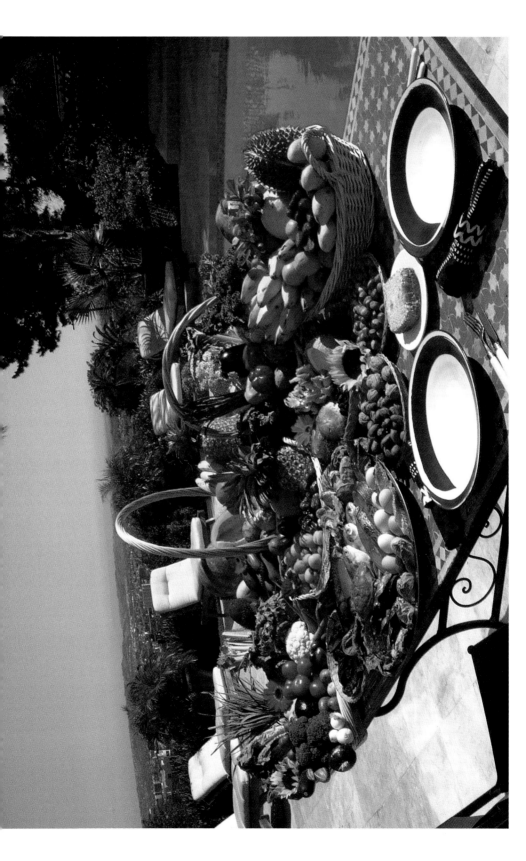

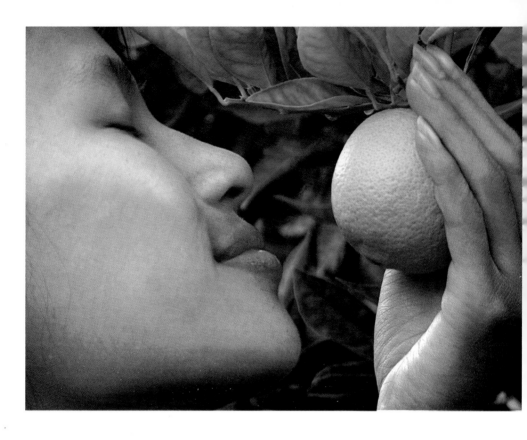

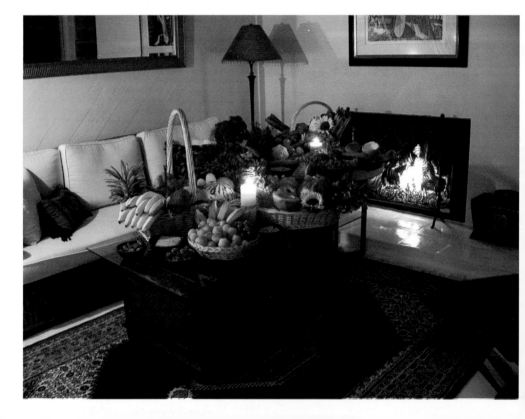

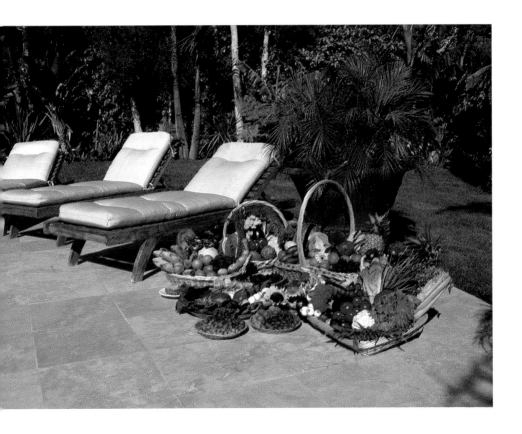
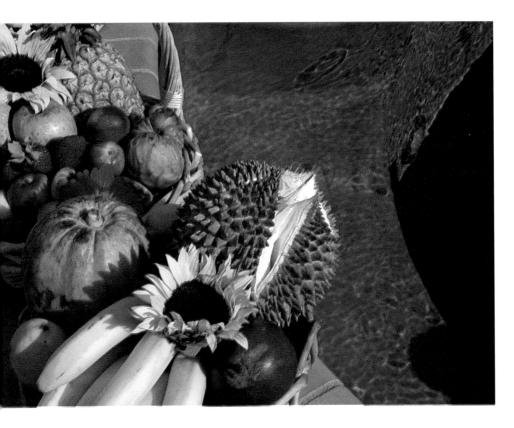

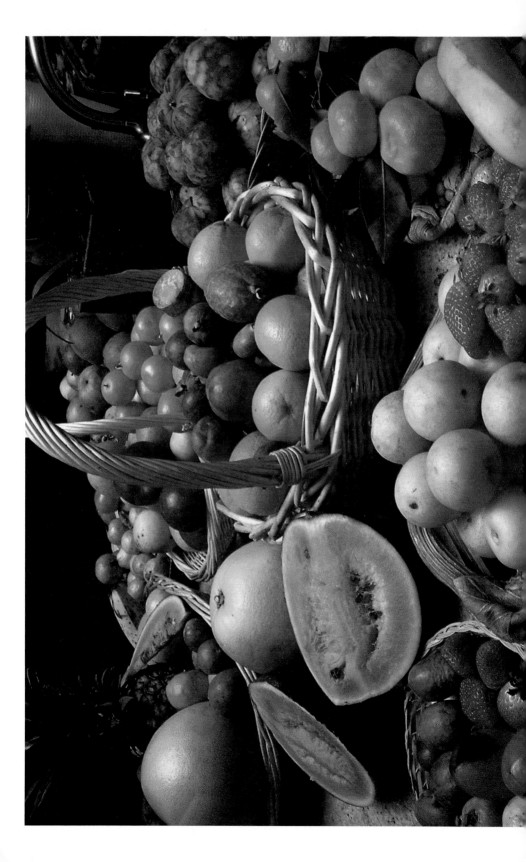

The case of Julie, a one-year-old girl, is a perfect example. During one of our daily Genefit Nutrition meals, Julie noticed an adult next to her eating apricots. The adult, Julie was carefully observing, was enjoying his apricots so intensely that she thought, "those apricots must be amazingly good." So, when she thought no one was watching, she took an apricot and put it into her mouth. Unfortunately, her body didn't need the apricot and so the taste was bad. She frowned and spat it out. Then she concluded that she probably grabbed a bad fruit and took another apricot, hoping the flavor would be better. Again, the taste was bad. She repeated the experiment eight times before she let go of the idea of having apricots that day. Her body simply didn't need them. Once she accepted that fact, she took an apricot and handed it to the person who was enjoying them.

For most of us who are less fortunate than Julie, the processed food paradigm began at birth, or even before, with nine months in our mother's body. As children, we receive hours of daily training in the relationship of food and pleasure. Unfortunately, when eating processed foods our reality of what pleasure is will be distorted and confused. Instead of the true sense of smell or taste, for example, a child will choose from an expectation or a prediction of what a food will taste like. With cooked or otherwise altered food, the taste and smell do not change. A cake or candy will taste as good today as it did yesterday. Thus, a child learns that he or she can predict or desire a reality and have it. In the beginning the desire is pleasure, even if the body is saying it is harmful.

As the child grows into adulthood the consequences of this training become more and more apparent. Paranoia, frustration, and apathy become more and more common as the child's desires of reality are not satisfied. The intellect tries even harder to get reality to obey, but the feeling that life is a struggle becomes inevitable. This confusion between desire and reality can be seen in many areas of life. Patricia's relationships end in disappointments as she is unable to get her men to be the way she wants them. Tom predicts that his life will be a certain way. At age forty he has a nervous breakdown after he loses his job. He feels frustrated, disappointed, and depressed. The mismatch between reality and desires can even lead to feelings of persecution, e.g., "Life is against me," "There is no justice in the world." In the old paradigm, Tom didn't learn to recognize his instincts, but grew up with the illusion that intellect can and should fulfill all of his desires. Psychiatric hospitals, and a society that needs substances to cope, illustrate the casualties of this aberrant training.

During early childhood, the first apprehensions of the surrounding environment influence the developing structures of the brain. The first impressions set brain development in one way or another, directly depending on the nature of those first perceptions. This is true for parental images and for acquiring perception of the laws of gravity as objects are seen falling. It is also true for gustatory experiences. Since they are the first, most powerful pleasure experiences of early childhood, they all make an imprint in a child's brain. After only a few meals with "solid" food, a child will have affirmations written in the subconscious, such as "baby food is good," or the opposite, "carrot juice is bad." Depending on how and under what circumstances those first experiences occurred, a child will build an inner representation, or referential, of the gustatory world surrounding him. Food preferences will become more and more distinct meal after meal. There is nothing wrong with experiences imprinting on the subconscious memory. It is a natural process. The problem does not come from the process itself; it comes from the nature of the environment we have artificially created. The inner referential coming from processed food is that of, figuratively speaking, a "frozen world." Since the taste is the same every time one eats a given food, and the level of pleasure is completely predictable, the relationship to that given food is static. It is "frozen" in place for all processed food, whether it was inscribed into memory in a negative or positive way. As you would expect with unprocessed food, since the taste is constantly changing and pleasure is proportionate to the body's constantly changing needs, the referential a child on Genefit Nutrition integrates is the referential of an ever-changing world. First impressions cannot be fixed in the same way. Laws cannot hold as absolute truth because they are constantly challenged by new gustatory perceptions. A pineapple might taste good sometimes and bad at others. For the mind, there are no static rules of taste. A child experiencing a taste change for the first time naturally integrates it, certainly by the time the food starts burning his tongue.

A person who eats instinctively would not expect a food to taste the same today as it did yesterday. The senses of taste and smell continually change depending on the person's physical needs. Nothing is "good" or "bad," and the mind is not compulsively anticipating the repetition of past pleasures.

How, then, do people who eat instinctively get pleasure? They learn to truly use their senses; to cooperate with their body; to be present and questioning in each new situation. In this true medium of interaction with the universe, change is neither traumatic nor to be feared. Change is a natural part of the experience of life. Children eating instinctively will be familiar, from an early age, with feelings of profound satisfaction and pleasure. As they learn the parameters of being in the physical world they will develop an underlying confidence and certainty in themselves and their abilities. The instinct and the intellect cooperate, interacting with the environment, people, circumstances, and life — dancing, not fighting.

When eating instinctively, the manner of choosing food, the awareness of the food as we eat, and the awareness of alliesthesial responses are all different from the processed food scenario. Consequently, eating instinctively, and the changes associated with it, can bring us face to face with fixed ways of thinking and being. These deep underlying differences are the main source of interference in any decision to bring about change.

The best response to an ever-changing world is interrogation. The gustatory referential of a processed food world is based on affirmations, presumptions, and prejudices. The gustatory referential of the unprocessed food world is based on receptiveness, interrogation, and openness. For a child, early gustatory experiences with unprocessed food make a huge difference. If those first experiences are truly instinctual, and for this they have to occur in a nutritional-instinct-friendly food environment, a child will develop trust in the nutritional instinct before rational thinking develops. In contrast, when olfactory and gustatory alliesthesia cannot be experienced, a child has no chance to build confidence in his own instinct, and when rational thinking comes to the surface, the mind will try to compensate for the past and present discomfort and symptoms that processed foods created. As an adult, the person will then grasp at all kinds of nutritional guidelines to recreate the sensation of security lost because of the absence of instinctual guidance. Analytic pathways will become overemphasized at the expense of instinctive built-in knowledge.

The traditional way we humans evaluate and process food biochemically in our bodies has thus been studied far more assiduously in laboratories than out in the real world we live in. Much has been learned about oxidants, hormones, fibers, amino acids, etc. New biochemical entities, and new types of old ones, are turning up daily. So much information has been accumulated, in fact, including so much that is seemingly contradictory, that by now, we can hardly even use it without some kind of nutritional philosophy or system as a guide. The practice of Genefit Nutrition might qualify as a philosophy too, except that the mechanisms of genetic adaptation to foods and the nutritional instinct developed long before the neurological mechanisms of brains fit for "thought."

Gustatory and olfactory alliesthesia is a tiny detail, overlooked by professionals in nutritional sciences, which changes the way a child relates to the world. It will also change the way you relate to the world, if you practice Genefit Nutrition long enough to reverse your former conditioning. In order to focus on your instinct, you must let go of what has become fixed, mainly back in early childhood. Genefit Nutrition is not a change of diet like any other. It requires and supports a psychological deconditioning.

People on Genefit Nutrition become accustomed to the notion that opinions appropriately change as conditions change. Fixed prejudices become unnatural. Of course, we all know, in theory, that flexibility in our opinions is sensible, but then in real life how many of us remember it? With Genefit Nutrition, you will experience it in your own body every day. As you become accustomed to your changing experience with food, you will soon notice changes in the way you relate to people around you and in the way you conduct your life. You will experience a real suppleness of the mind. Intuition and self-confidence will strengthen. Suddenly, the usual classifications of people will start to crumble. And when there is nothing else left to hold onto, only interrogation will remain. Interrogation is the surrendering of the mind to the reality we live in, and the body is part of that reality. Letting go to a complete inner state of interrogation produces the very particular state sought by many spiritual traditions. This state is often the ultimate object of meditation. The mystical question "Who am I?" may naturally start with the simple question, "What does my body need at this moment?" This awareness naturally extends to other situations, in addition to eating experiences, and becomes more and more a permanent state of mind. Be prepared. Genefit Nutrition is much more than a diet. It is a profound, life-changing experience, because it reconnects you with the deepest layers of yourself, away from opinions, representations, prejudices, and social personality. Once you have experienced it, you won't look at the world the same way ever again.

Eating by instinct is really the simplest way there is. We need only trust our own nature and that of our foods. Infants and children will do so spontaneously, if allowed to. Adults, educated in ways aimed at developing the intellect, may need to put forth an effort to unlearn what they think they know, to make room for sensations and feelings. We may stumble at first, and perhaps make mistakes. But merely starting gives confidence, and leads, ultimately (and in a surprisingly short time), to a degree of satisfaction in being alive that dead foods and prescribed ways of eating cannot provide.

In summary, is there any better metaphor that can be given to illustrate the discussion in this chapter than the following quote by George Bernard Shaw?

> The only person I really trust is my tailor. He takes my measurements every time I see him.

NINE

Peace of Mind

EXPERIMENT 6

Repeat Experiment 4 with your friends or family. Make everyone smell at least five different fruits with closed eyes. After everybody has chosen his or her fruit, you will notice that different people choose different fruits. People's needs vary depending on many internal and external factors. Each individual's nutritional instinct is matching these personal needs as closely as possible to the optimum food, within the given parameters.

ALCOHOL IS A SMALL MOLECULE that easily crosses the blood/brain barrier. When consumed in beverages such as liquors, beer, or wine, it enters the brain and alters perception and behavior. After a certain quantity has been consumed, people simply become drunk. Similarly, neuroactive substances, such as caffeine, enter the brain and modify the perception and behavior of the individual who ingested them. For example, when someone under the influence of caffeine encounters a stressful situation, he can easily become abnormally irritated. Most of us have experienced both of these phenomena. Similar signs of chemically induced neuroactivity also result from the consumption of abnormal molecules in processed foods.

Except for a few isolated studies, the neurological mechanisms involving our responses to chemicals in processed foods have never been explored, for the good reason that their existence was never seriously recognized. Most medical researchers to date have assumed that denatured foods were normal for humans and so have remained unaware of their effects. Even when the existence of neuroactive and neurotoxic chemicals in daily processed food was sometimes suspected, neurologists most often thought that the blood/brain barrier would be impermeable enough to hinder them from entering the brain.

From an empirical standpoint, Genefit Nutrition will give you an opportunity to observe how these chemicals affect us. If you later revert to a dinner of melted cheese on whole-wheat toast and soup, and discover that shortly thereafter you have become inexplicably anxious, tense, impatient, irritable, and stressed, the phenomenon will no longer be unexplainable. Surprisingly, the effects of processed food on the brain are widely underestimated, and yet, we don't have to dig very far to comprehend the mechanisms involved.

A protein present in wheat by-products, called gluten, has been proven to be highly neuroactive. The presence of gluten in the food palette is enough to produce schizophrenic symptoms in people prone to schizophrenia. Casein, a protein contained in cow's milk, has been found to play a role in autism.[1-2] Other studies have shown a clear link between processed food and hyperactivity in children.[3] Molecules coming from processed food are not only neuroactive, affecting behavior and perception in the present, but also neurotoxic, damaging the brain's functions over time. Abnormal molecules, such as Maillard molecules, have a tendency to accumulate in the brain and play a role in pathologies like Alzheimer's disease, which, by the way, affects primarily elderly people among whom the accumulation has had a lifetime to take place.[4] Of all the organs in the body, the brain has been widely recognized to be the most sensitive to chemical changes. So why should there be any doubt that new chemical substances contained in processed food can have an effect on the way we think, act, and perceive the world?

Differences in behavior and perception, when switching from a traditional diet to eating by instinct, were observed very soon after the discovery of the nutritional instinct. Most people who volunteered to eat instinctively at the time noticed a difference in the way they felt and acted. The most astonishing and convincing results came from the animal world. Since animals do not have the same inhibitory mechanisms we have, the results are clear and free from cultural influences. In the past, a small team of researchers investigating the benefits of an instinctive way of eating used to have rats in their laboratory. These rats were subject to the same treatment as many humans were in evolutionary history: switching back and forth between a processed and an unprocessed food environment. At that time, there was an interest in the impact of different food environments on animals. Those who are familiar with the behavior of rats probably know that rats have an instinct pushing them to devour each other when forced into overcrowded spaces. Eating each other is the rat's natural response to overpopulation. We should consider ourselves pretty lucky to have evolved, don't you think?

The rats in this laboratory were fed natural, unprocessed food most of the time. They practiced the "rat's version" of Genefit Nutrition. Occasionally, processed food was introduced in order to observe the effects on their bodies and their behavior. Typically, two males fed strictly unprocessed foods would be living in a cage big enough for them to tolerate each other. Each one stayed in its little corner of the cage, permitting a somewhat peaceful cohabitation. When processed food, such as bread or cheese, was fed, it was not uncommon to find one and a half rats in the cage the next day; one had partially eaten the other. This experiment shows that processed food alters the tolerance of rats to crowding. The natural instinct to devour each other is triggered differently under the exact same space parameters, depending on whether they are fed processed food or unprocessed food.

The first time this phenomenon was observed, it was by accident. Related questions about human behavior naturally came to mind. Can we extrapolate the result of the above experiment to human beings? Even if we don't possess the exact same instincts as rats, we still have instincts driving us, whether we recognize them as such or not. Aggressiveness, for example, clearly has an instinctual origin we have inherited from the animal world. What happens in our world today is not always a model of psychological balance. Examples of aggressiveness can be found in the persistent religious conflicts in various parts of the world, random violence in large cities, terrorist activity, etc. They are not really what we can call the best behavior in the best possible world. This is not to say that Genefit Nutrition can free us from all conflicts and violence. As for our rats, even if humans might have an instinctual aggressiveness, which can, by the way, serve a purpose, this aggressiveness can then become widely emphasized under unnatural eating conditions. It will then not necessarily follow a strictly natural action-reaction pattern, but might, to a certain extent, be chemically auto-induced.

To understand what triggers such phenomena, let's consider basic brain function. The brain is a network of trillions of neurons interacting with each other. Neurons and nerve cells of the body communicate with one another through synapses that function like junction boxes, collecting little electric signals from incoming neurons and passing them on to others. Signals travel from one neuron to another as we speak, think, walk, or read. Electrical impulses occurring in the brain are chemically generated by natural processes, which are controlled by neurons. A synapse will transmit (i.e., pass an impulse downstream to the next cell in the circuit) only if enough upstream (incoming) pulses are present to produce a charge powerful enough to set it off. A synapse's minimal transmitting threshold can be modified by drugs. Tranquilizers raise them, so that more input is needed for output to be produced. Stimulants have the opposite effect. Any foreign neuroactive molecule entering the brain can hinder electric impulses from being fired or abnormally amplify them. In addition, some neuronal circuits include a feedback system, which, among other things, helps adjust the strength of the outgoing signal. When the incoming signal passing from the first neuron to the second neuron is too strong, as may happen when it is amplified by the effect of abnormal molecules, the electrical signal going through the feedback system is also strengthened. As a result, the whole system starts looping abnormally, as happens when a microphone gets too close to the speakers, creating that typical whistle noise commonly called "the Larsen effect." In this case, emotions and thoughts can become auto-amplified and self-perpetuating. If you ever had that song you couldn't get out of your mind, even though you wanted to, you can relate to that phenomenon. It never happens under Genefit Nutrition eating conditions when the bloodstream is clear from abnormal molecules.

Thanks to observations of a significant number of people on Genefit Nutrition, we now have a standard of comparison that leads us to infer that abnormal food either causes so-called "normal" thresholds to be abnormally low, or creates an abnormally high level of internal nervous stimulation. The brain can then enter a state of self-reflexive feedback, leading to thoughts, emotions, and actions having little or no relation to reality.

> Moreover, I have evidence that the polypeptides that develop during the digestion of cereal grains are trigger factors, and it has been observed that the activity of some of them is comparable to that of endorphins. This . . . is based on three observations:

1) There seems to be a strong correlation between the changes in behavior of schizophrenics when first admitted to the hospital and the changes that occur with wheat intake, or wheat and barley intake (multiple regression).

2) The kind of diet and epidemiological data leads one to conclude that the risk of morbid schizophrenia is greater if an individual eats a lot of wheat (and barley), slightly lower for rice-eaters, and still lower with individuals whose staple grains include corn on the cob, millet, and barley.

3) Clinical observation suggests that allergies to gluten (coeliac disease) and schizophrenia are genetically linked; such an assertion requires formal confirmation through in-depth studies of families showing signs of coeliac disease.

These facts, as well as others, impelled us to confirm whether eating wheat gluten again was enough to revive all the disorders that had subsided on a 100 percent cereal-grain-free and milk-free diet.

That was the case . . . . It was shown that there was endorphic activity in the peptidic metabolites in milk casein, and in corn and barley gluten, as well as very strong activity in wheat gluten (T.C. Dohan, *Schizophrenia and Dietary Neuroactive Peptides*, Department of Molecular Biology, Pennsylvania Psychiatric Institute, in *The Lancet*, May 12, 1979, p. 1031).

Two classes of denatured (and in this case, unnatural) food seem to contribute most severely to creating altered behavior. The first is cereals, particularly wheat. The second is milk and its by-products. For millions of years, those categories of food were not on the human menu; they are recent innovations. Most books on nutrition claim that whole-wheat bread is better food than white-flour bread, since it contains fibers, minerals, and vitamins that refined flour has lost. But it also contains more gluten, which wreaks even more havoc with our nervous system than refined wheat does. If you have been eating grains, particularly whole grains, you will probably notice, almost at once, when you give them up that you are less keyed up. The same prediction goes for milk.

In some situations, removing milk from the diet can result in dramatic improvements in behavior, especially hyperactive children. In four out of five children, aged six to fifteen, found to be sensitive to milk, all reported "markedly positive" improvement when milk was completely eliminated from the diet (Alexander Schauss, *Diet, Crime and Delinquency*, Parker House, Berkeley, 1984).

Chimpanzees have been observed to occasionally kill members of a neighbor group, even in an unprocessed food environment. Same-species murder among mammals exists under natural conditions, as the chimpanzees' behavior indicates. For humans, on the other hand, it is very interesting to note that no trace of organized war has ever been found before the advent of food processing. War campaigns, such as those conducted later by the Greeks and Romans, do not seem to have occurred before cooking became common usage. No crushed bones from earlier times, which would indicate that rival tribes fought each other, have ever been found. If such behavior had been widespread, it is most likely that we would have found traces of it. Signs of violence found back in the Paleolithic era were among Neanderthals. At the verge of extinction, during the long winters when food was scarce, they eventually became cannibals. Other traces of violence on human skeletons were caused by wild animals. The skeleton of a child has been found in Africa with two holes in the skull, resulting from the dentition of a lion. Man was hunted before he became a hunter.

Changes in the food environment, which occurred at the beginning of agriculture, are probably not enough to explain the appearance of organized war; other sociological factors were probably involved. For example, clan possessiveness over agricultural land and products may have been an unnatural source of tensions; or changes in the social structure coming along with big civilizations may have inspired killing behavior. On the other hand, repeated experiments have brought us enough elements to ask ourselves a fundamental question: How would we reason, act, and perceive the world if we completely avoided artificial molecules made neuroactive by processing in our daily food?

Past and present observations of both humans and animals brought us to the same conclusion: chemicals in processed food significantly alter the way we think, act, and perceive the world. When a family practicing Genefit Nutrition for some time introduces a single processed food into its diet, the level of conflicts and tensions unavoidably starts to rise. The extraordinary peaceful state acquired thanks to Genefit Nutrition becomes disrupted. Commonplace issues that are naturally handled without any problem suddenly become troublesome with the introduction of just one processed food. Impatience, irritability, and aggressiveness become amplified as abnormal molecules enter the bloodstream.

Of course, an aggressive person will not be transformed into an angel overnight because of Genefit Nutrition, and a person on Genefit Nutrition will not turn into a demon when eating processed food. But comparatively, there is clearly a significant difference in behavior after switching between food environments. And the difference is big enough to have a major impact on social interaction and relationships. Nowadays, because food processing has become so omnipresent, and modern, civilized people have never lived long enough within a strictly unprocessed food environment to experience this difference, the effects of abnormal molecules on our behavior are still largely underestimated.

With Genefit Nutrition, the brain returns to its original way of functioning. Chemically induced emotions and behaviors disappear. When practiced in a very precise manner, Genefit Nutrition spontaneously produces a meditation-like state of mind, which is prevented by diets consisting of processed food. The mind stream can be interrupted by will without applying any meditation technique. You will experience this unique state of mind if you apply the principles of Genefit Nutrition consistently over longer periods of time. You will be surprised by the impact food can have on the brain and how things as fundamental as world peace are dependent on whatever is on our plates.

NOTES

1. S. Lucarelli , T. Frediani, A.M. Zingoni, F. Ferruzzi, O. Giardini, F. Quintieri, M. Barbato, P. D'Eufemia, E. Cardi, "Food allergy and infantile autism." Panminerva Med 1995 Sep;37(3):137-41.

2. D. O'Banion, B. Armstrong, R.A. Cummings., J. Stange,"Disruptive behavior: a dietary approach." *Autism Child Schizophr* 1978 Sep;8(3):325-37.

3. J. Breakey, "The role of diet and behaviour in childhood." *Paediatr Child Health* 1997 Jun;33(3):190-4.

4. M.A. Smith, S. Taneda, P.L. Richey, S. Miyata, S.D. Yan, D. Stern, L.M. Sayre, V.M. Monnier, G. Perry,"Advanced Maillard reaction end products are associated with Alzheimer disease pathology" *Proc Natl Acad Sci USA* 1994 Jun 7;91(12):5710-4.

— TEN —

Foods that Poison
and Symptoms that Heal

HOW CAN WE EXPLAIN OUR DRIVE, unique among living things, to convert whatever natural thing we touch into something that never existed before? In order to transform our food, we learned to use fire, coals and hot stones, skewers, leaf wrappings, pots and pans, covers, pressure cookers, gas and electric and microwave ovens, and infrared radiators. Cooking is, by far, the most effective and radical way to modify food. Heat speeds up the movements of the food's atoms, disturbs their electrostatic bonds, and accelerates their interactions. It creates new chemical compounds and molecules that did not exist before.

However, cooking is not generally thought of as chemistry. It is not called a science. It is known as an art. In the kitchen, it is legitimate to add a spoonful of X, a pinch of Y, a handful of Z, and a cup of Q to roughly two pounds of K, and raise the temperature to medium for an hour or so. Any laboratory chemist who operated in these terms would be fired on the spot.

Cooking can be regulated, as it is in assembly-line kitchens, so that each batch of cooked product contains carefully measured amounts of the same types of ingredients. This may ensure uniform quality, but the manufacturer will be eager to point out that the aroma arising from each and every one of his million cans a day is due to somebody's art. The only difference between a kitchen and a laboratory is that in the latter we know what's going on. Whatever the outcome, we know it came from specific compounds mixed under specific conditions at known temperatures. In a kitchen, however, we simply have no means of analyzing the chemical compounds produced by the interactions between the proteins, acids, fats, starches, salts, oils, onions, tomatoes, garlic, salt, pepper, bay leaf, and, in some cases, beef (whose tissues probably also contain hormones, vaccines, fertilizer and pesticide residues). Then we bring it all together and simmer for an hour or two. We may feel, with some justification, that the type of analysis that concerns us in the kitchen is of another kind. If it smells good, if it tastes good, that's what counts. We may take care to undercook our vegetables, so as not to destroy the vitamins (and then take a few synthetic ones just in case), but generally, our precautions end there.

Since we have eaten cooked foods all our lives, they seem as natural as the air we breathe. We do not link symptoms to chemical changes, because we can hardly conceive that they even took place at all. But we are not genetically prepared for them. While our bodies can manufacture only a limited number of enzymes to break down ingested molecular structures to render them usable, our culinary ingenuity is capable of creating unlimited numbers of new ones, which are unknown to our biochemical makeup.

Very few scientists were ever concerned about toxic compounds in processed food. Some time at the beginning of the last century, an American chemical engineer named Maillard discovered that the simple act of cooking a potato in boiling water produces 420 new molecules not present in the original, unprocessed potato. He concluded that when a food is exposed to heat over a specific temperature, because of the molecular agitation, carbohydrate and protein chains break and combine randomly. Today, we call those molecules Maillard molecules. What were only 420 for a cooked potato can become millions or even billions of different molecules in complex recipes. The possible new chemical compounds so produced are virtually limitless. Maillard reactions occurring in a kitchen are not controlled in any way. They originate from chaos, so it is impossible to completely foresee what types of new chemical substances will be produced in a given recipe. This is, by the way, not the concern of the cook; only taste is.

To illustrate this point, fry an egg on a dry skillet and watch the albumin turn white. You may wonder, what is happening to its molecular structure? No one really knows. Every time we ever watched an egg turn white, we were dealing with "cooking," not "chemistry," so the question had never been seriously asked, not even in our largest research institutions.

Now, cook another egg, this time breaking the membrane between yolk and white and scrambling them together. Here, we are creating even more complex interactions at high temperature, which would never occur in nature. What dynamic structures are they producing, and how will our bodies handle them? Once you have learned to eat instinctively with unprocessed food exclusively, you will be able to answer this question easily: with physical discomfort and pain!

And just once more, for good measure: let us cook our next egg with some oil on the skillet, some pieces of last night's potatoes, and some cheese, salt, and pepper mixed in. This time, how many new compounds of unknown structure did we create? As surprising as it sounds, nobody knows. But, if now we only brown the potatoes:

> As far back as 1916, Maillard proved that the brown pigments and polymers that occur in pyrolysis (chemical breakdown by heat alone) . . . are yielded after prior reaction of an amino acid group with the carbonyl group of sugars. Though apparently simple, this reaction is, in fact, highly complex, iterating in a spate of successive reactions and forming melanoidins, which are brown pigments that impart a typical color to whatever part of a food has endured higher temperatures. The number of substances generated as a result is most impressive, yielding endless chains of new molecules: ketones, esters, aldehydes, ethers, volatile alcohols, and non-volatile heterocycles, etc.
>
> These innumerable substances coalesce into a complex compound and are endowed with differing biological and chemical attributes: they are toxic, aromatic, peroxidizing, anti-oxidizing, and possibly mutagenic and carcinogenic (DNA fractures can be oncogenic), or even anti-mutagenic and anti-carcinogenic. This to say that heating causes widespread disruption in the natural order of molecules. The research work backing up this article evidenced over 50 pyrolytic substances in broiled potatoes, most of which originated from pyroseines and thiazole. However, there remain, all in all, some 400 by-products to identify (Professor R. Derache, "Pyrolysis and risks of toxicity" *Cahiers de nutrition et de dietetique* [*Diet and Nutrition Journal*], 1982, p 39).

As already mentioned in the beginning of this book, further research has confirmed that some of those new molecules are:

- toxic (produces body intoxication)
- carcinogenic (produces cancer cells)
- mutagenic (disturbs DNA replication)
- neurotoxic (affects brain functions)
- antigenic (involved in autoimmune diseases)

Among the molecular abnormalities that have been identified so far we count: oxidants, free radicals, ketones, esters, aldehydes, volatile alcohols, heterocycles, pyroseines, thiazole, premelanoidins, glycation endproducts, melanoidins, and many others.

Maillard molecules are not the only category of new chemical substances the body has been confronted by since the invention of food processing. Even though some have been identified, there are numerous others that have not yet been taken into consideration. Maillard end products alone can be found in any food exposed to a certain temperature. They are basically everywhere culinary art is applied.

It is not our aim to alarm anyone, except about the state of our ignorance. Our best-known writers in medicine, nutrition, and dietetics usually fail to distinguish between raw and cooked food, except in limited terms of nutrients lost or destroyed. And when nutritional value is discussed, it is not always clear what values are being referred to. Put another way: when a child gets lost, he knows where he is. It's his parents who don't. When we "lose" nutrients in the pot, it's not that they've vanished into thin air (although some volatile ones may effectively be carried away), but rather that they've combined with others to make new kinds of molecules. They've gone where we can't find them any longer. A food's "nutritional value" may, in effect, be destroyed or "lost," but it is its value that is so affected, not the molecules themselves. They do not cease to exist, but become transformed in ways neither our laboratories nor our enzymes can identify.

> In general terms the premelanoidins formed during the first stages of roasting meat are not digestible and even have negative effects on the digestibility of the unaltered proteins and on protein efficiency ("Consequences Nutritionnelles de la Cuisson par les Micro-Ondes" [*Nutritional Consequences of Cooking with Microwaves*], Araudo & Sorbier, Ibid.).

Just for emphasis, let us briefly take a look at the kind of cooking (i.e., chemistry) done, not in skillets, but in commercial kitchen-factories whose products fill so much of our supermarket shelf space. We will consider just one product, a popular type of cookie. The recipe is somewhat different from the one familiar to Girl Scouts; it contains, at the outset, no natural ingredients at all — except possibly whole eggs (if they were actually added straight from the shell, which is doubtful). According to the label, the cookies contained before being processed:

> Cottonseed oil, soybean oil, beef or pork fat, unbleached flour, Vitamin A, Vitamin D, ferrous sulphate, thiamine, niacin, riboflavin, sugar, skim milk, cocoa, dextrose, egg yolks, soya flour, starch, sodium acid pyrophosphate, baking soda, sodium aluminum phosphate, fumaric acid, salt, toasted ground wheat, rye flour, corn flour, potato flour, whole eggs, egg whites, guar gum, karaya gum, dextrin, lecithin, polysorbate 60, sodium stearol-2-lactylate, sodium caseinate, mono- and dyglycerides, propylene glycol mono and diesters, whey, spice, artificial colors, artificial flavor, and corn syrup.

Merely baking this mixture would produce recompounded chemical structures of indescribable complexity that are completely alien to our digestive systems. But in the factory, even further denaturation occurs. In order to increase its market appeal, the mixture will be texturized by a process that deliberately causes the macromolecules in the ingredients to lose their native organization and structure. The batter will be sent to a preconditioner to be precooked, then extruded through a device where it will again be heated by mechanical torsion and possibly even injected steam

> ". . . which transforms it into a viscous, plasticized material whose denatured molecules can recombine at their exposed electrostatic, hydrogen, covalent and ionic bonding sites . . ." (J.W. Harper, "Extrusion Texturization of Foods," *Food Technology*, Vol. 40, No. 3, 1986).

We are incapable of even imagining, let alone determining by analysis, all the kinds of molecular novelties such methods produce. We should only marvel that the product is labeled "food."

All of this is to say that cooking and chemistry might usefully be thought of together. Raising the temperature of a food changes its molecular structure. At the least, we will eat it to excess, because denatured food will not trigger an alliesthesial response to protect us from eating more than we need, leading to a toxic overload. But we will also be ingesting toxic compounds the food did not contain in its original state.

There is great significance for humans in the results of a unique nutritional experiment that was carried out to compare the effects of raw versus cooked food on cats (and incidentally, on plants). The results carry heavy implications for human well-being, but have largely been ignored by the medical profession. They corroborate the Genefit Nutrition thesis that no animal can, without ill effect, ingest food its genetic code is not prepared to metabolize. The study, carried out over a ten-year period in the 1930s and 1940s, compared the health, skeletal, and dental development of two populations of cats. One group was fed essentially raw meat scraps, the other cooked meat, with raw milk for both groups (later experiments reversed this to raw milk for one group and cooked milk for others, with raw meat for both):

CATS ON RAW MEAT DIET

Over their life spans they prove resistant to infections, to fleas and various other parasites, and show no signs of allergies. In general they are gregarious, friendly and predictable in their behavior patterns. When dropped as much as six feet to test their coordination they always land on their feet and come back for more "play." These cats produce one homogeneous generation after another with the average weight of the kitten at birth being 119 grams. Miscarriages are rare and the litters average five kittens with the mother cat nursing her young without difficulty.

CATS ON COOKED MEAT DIET

Heart problems; nearsightedness and farsightedness; underactivity of the thyroid or inflammation of the thyroid gland; infections of the kidney, of the liver, of the testes, of the ovaries and of the bladder; arthritis and inflammation of the joints; inflammation of the nervous system with paralysis and meningitis — all occur commonly in these cooked meat fed cats. Cooked meat fed cats show much more irritability. Some females are even dangerous to handle. . . .the males on the other hand are more docile, even to the point of being unaggressive and their sex interest is slack or perverted . . . Vermin and intestinal parasites abound. Skin lesions and allergies appear frequently and are progressively worse from one generation to the next . . . Abortion in pregnant females is common, running about 25 percent in the first cooked meat generation to about 70 percent in the second. Deliveries are generally difficult with many females dying in labor . . . . The average weight of the kittens is 100 grams, 19 grams less than the raw meat nurtured kittens (Francis M. Pottenger, Jr., *Pottenger's Cats*, The Price-Pottenger Nutrition Foundation, San Diego, 1983).

Cow's milk in any form is not an original food for cats, only for calves. Experiments performed on several generations of cats within a Genefit Nutritional reference frame showed that cats fed strictly unprocessed food without milk have odorless feces. Blindfolded people, who smelled those feces without knowing what it was, reported an odor of cardboard or mushroom, at most. As soon as milk is introduced, the same cat's feces developed the usual strong and well-known odor right after the first consumption. For the cat feces to turn odorless again, it takes about the same amount of time as the amount of time during which milk was consumed. Healthwise, Pottenger's cats apparently did relatively well on cow's milk, as long as it was raw, but unfortunately, he did not explore the effects of a totally milk-free diet on his animals, except by accident, without remarking upon the total absence of milk:

> Kittens in which deficiency is established by an inadequate diet show stigmata throughout their lives. If deficient kittens are allowed to live in the open and feed upon rats, mice, birds, gophers and other food natural to the cat, they will show a certain degree of correction in their deficiencies.

In fact, a partial correction of many deficiencies and a healing of disease symptoms is exactly what happens to humans when they eat exclusively unprocessed food — when they "forage" by instinct among a variety of raw, unprocessed foods. We should not really be surprised.

In another study showing the effects of instinctive feeding, a group of guinea pigs was initially fed a diet of rolled and cracked grain with supplements of cod liver oil and field-dried alfalfa. In a short time, they showed loss of hair, paralysis, and high litter mortality, with an increase in pneumonia, diarrhea, and other deficiency symptoms. When fresh-cut green grass was introduced into their diet, they showed remarkable improvement. A few guinea pigs with severe diarrhea were allowed to run outside the pens to feed on growing grass and weeds. In less than thirty days, these animals showed even greater improvement than those receiving fresh-cut greens inside the pens. Their diarrhea stopped, their hair returned with a soft, shiny, velvety texture, and they healed and became well, with no recurrence of gastrointestinal upset or other ailments.[1]

The Pottenger experiments included a comparison of the effects on farm chickens that were free to eat worms, grasses, and weeds, with hatchery chickens, housed in wire pens and fed dry feeds. The former laid eggs with hard shells and deep-yellow yolks, from which husky, healthy chicks hatched. In contrast, hatchery chickens laid thin-shelled eggs with pale yolks, a large percentage of which failed to germinate when fertilized. The farm chickens contained twice as much calcium as the mass-produced ones.

In comparing the diets of farm and mass-produced chickens and of range and dry-fed lot cattle, we find that they all contain adequate amounts of fat, protein, carbohydrates, and minerals. The difference lies in the presence or absence of abnormal molecules, such as Maillard molecules. It is the absence of species-inappropriate or abnormal molecules in feed that appears to hold the balance between a healthy animal capable of reproducing healthy offspring and one that is unhealthy, having poor reproductive efficiency.

Pottenger did several experiments raising navy beans in separate plots of ground fertilized with the excreta of cats fed raw or cooked food. The plants were compared for germination rates, growth rates, size, and appearance. The raw-food excreta fertilized plants did well, while plants grown with cooked-food excreta fertilizer did poorly. The greatest contrast appeared in quality of the beans:

> RAW MEAT: These beans have a hard, white surface. Uniformity of size and plumpness of the beans distinguishes them from the beans of all other groups.

> COOKED MEAT: In this group, one-fourth of the beans are shriveled and yellow in color; the remainder are smooth and white. They also are more plump than the milk beans, but they are not as plump as the raw meat beans. They exhibit the peculiar oblong shape of the milk beans (Francis M. Pottenger, Jr., *Pottenger's Cats*, The Price-Pottenger Nutrition Foundation, San Diego, 1983).

It should be evident that when animals, man included, or plants ingest foods to which they are not adapted, abnormalities will occur. It should also be evident that the genetic code of each living organism is prepared to properly metabolize and make use only of the foods it is "familiar with" from the millions of years of its evolutionary past. But, we are not familiar with molecules to which the body hasn't had time to adapt. We are also not familiar with "vitamin C" and "vitamin B12" and "zinc" and "iron" and "calcium." Our bodies do indeed require some variable amounts of the molecules these verbal abstractions refer to. But we do not require them as isolated entities, packaged in separate bottles for marketing convenience. They are never separate in nature. The whole is more than the sum of its parts. A peach is more than "fructose" + "fiber" + "vitamin C" + "water," and we did not become genetically adapted to its analyzable parts. We evolved in relationship to the unified whole, fresh factor included.

> An analysis of a dead body and an analysis of a handful of soil will show them to both be composed of the same elements, but no one can mistake the flesh of a man for a handful of soil. An apple, too, is made up of the same elements as the soil, but we easily recognize the vast difference between this product of vital synthesis and the soil in our garden. (Herbert M. Shelton. *The Science and Fine Art of Food and Nutrition*, Natural Hygiene Press, Oldsmar, 1984.)

As zookeepers can testify, almost any wild animal fed denatured foods will quickly become sick and die, poisoned by unnatural molecules it is unable to process. On the other hand, digestively speaking, humans, hogs, and rats are the planet's most versatile species. Those "ambulatory garbage dumps" of the animal kingdom can eat practically any denatured food and somehow survive long enough to reproduce. Humans, along with the pigs and rats that eat their leftovers, are generally able to adjust for a period of time. At this point, it all depends on what we are looking for: survival, despite unnatural circumstances, or optimal health in a nutritional context that is truly natural for us. Shouldn't our intelligence be used to create a food environment that supports health instead of denaturing food, as is mostly the case?

The current medical notion of intoxication refers to poisoning the body with chemicals, drugs, and gasses, which are artificially produced for the most part, or bacteria, venom, or recognized toxic foods such as toadstools, spoiled meat, or accumulated metabolic wastes. Detoxification refers to eliminating these types of poisons or rendering them harmless. But the usual notion of toxic substances fails to take account of the alien (and demonstrably toxic) molecules contained in processed food. So, we are using the term intoxination to denote the unrecognized poisoning produced by the altered molecular structure of nonoriginal foods. We will occasionally refer to the poisons themselves as nutritional toxins, including all abnormal molecules food processing produces. A derived word, detoxination, will be used in reference to the elimination of nutritional toxins from the body. Detoxination often occurs in ways, and via channels, that are not recognized for what they are — a cleansing, health-restoring process. Consequently, the symptoms of detoxination are more often than not classified as symptoms of an illness, and efforts are made to suppress them, frequently with drugs. The medical intervention unfortunately halts the cleaning-out process and hinders the body's profound regeneration task. This may, in turn, cause other new symptoms to appear in the future (that again constitute detoxination phenomena, again not recognized as such) leading again to new attempts at suppression with drugs. A vicious cycle results, producing iatrogenic disease, that is, a disease caused by drugs.

Detoxination is a natural and necessary process that occurs spontaneously if not interfered with. Even though our prehistoric ancestors ate mostly unprocessed foods to which they were genetically adapted, they would also have been ingesting any number of things their bodies couldn't use and would need to eliminate, such as food that was not in a pristine original condition: plant food after a forest fire, or fallen fruit that had baked in the sun. Consequently, their genetic code necessarily included instructions for eliminating the toxins these less-than-perfect foods contained, just as ours does today. However, there is a major difference: the amount of abnormal molecules consumed accidentally was very little, compared to the ones consumed nowadays. Today, the daily load of new chemical substances entering the body is simply enormous, and they aren't related to what may have happened before the time food processing came into existence. At that time, any symptom associated with detoxination was probably nonexistent. Today, there are abundant, abnormal molecules in food, and the emunctory systems, which include liver, kidneys, intestines, bladder, skin, lungs, tongue, and mucous membranes, are overloaded. Unless detoxination is carefully regulated, the cleansing becomes troublesome.

If there is any doubt that we are daily ingesting huge amounts of unnatural chemical compounds, let us remember that the novel smells of cooked foods (among others) indicate the presence of novel molecules. Our olfactory system is extremely sensitive. In some cases, few molecules may suffice to trigger a smell sensation. And, surprising as it may seem, even though sophisticated laboratory instruments and procedures may be unable to detect these novel compounds, our noses usually can.

When diets are restricted to unprocessed foods only, in their original, unmodified state, human beings and animals carry practically no odors at all. Their urine, feces, sweat, breath, sputum, vaginal discharges, etc., barely smell. It is only when ingested substances are incompletely metabolized that they carry a significant odor. What this means, in practical terms, is that after eating only unprocessed foods instinctively for a time, you will not have bad breath, your unwashed feet will not stink, and your excrement and urine will be close to odorless.

Let us try to better understand what it means if a person does carry odors. Assume you have been practicing Genefit Nutrition long enough to become basically free of odors. Then, suddenly odors reappear. If no other factor changes the only reasons can be:

1. either you are discharging (detoxinating) unnatural wastes from some nonoriginal food you just ate, or
2. you are flushing out (detoxinating) remnants from nonoriginal food you ate in the past.

When this happens, your odors will tell you what it is you just ate — or what it was that had accumulated in your body from whatever you ate years ago, or regularly over many years, that is now finding its way out.

For example, let us say you have been regularly eating by instinct and have become free of odors. Then, on an impulse, one evening you eat some roasted peanuts instead of raw ones. For a few days, your perspiration and general body odor will smell exactly the way the roasted peanuts smelled before you ate them, unchanged. And once the roasted peanut molecules have been eliminated, you will become odorless again. The body had no use for the "roasted" molecules, since they are not part of our native dietary spectrum. So, they were eliminated right away.

When an unprocessed, natural, genetically appropriate food is eaten, its molecules are first broken down (catabolized) by acids, enzymes, and bacteria, in the stomach and intestinal tract, and are then rebuilt (anabolized) into molecules (metabolites), usable by the cells. The process involves long chemical chain reactions, analogous to a series of chambers behind locked doors, where each molecule is like a key that must be correctly reshaped to fit the next lock if it is to pass through each successive chamber, all the way to the end. However, when food has been denatured, it is like a misshapen key that will open only a few doors and consequently is unable to go through the entire digestive process.

Because of the genetic nonadaptation to roasted peanuts, human beings do not possess the enzymatic or other digestive wherewithal to metabolize them. If humans possessed the enzymes to metabolize roasted peanut molecules, they would not smell anymore after having gone through the digestive and metabolic processes. They do smell on their way out, because some molecules contained in the roasted peanuts will have been either only partly altered or not altered at all. They will sometimes consist of intermediary (semi-cooked) compounds that a human cannot break down completely and can only use in part. Some of these compounds, because they are alien only to a degree, may get started through the metabolic process and then get stuck along the way.

What happens then is that even big, undigested molecules cross the intestinal barrier, entering the bloodstream and lymphatic system. The uptake from the intestine of big, undigested molecules or macromolecules has been scientifically recognized as a natural process in itself. But, even if this process is natural, some of the molecules ingested are not. The reason the body opens the door to what can potentially be harmful molecules currently remains unknown.

> Although the majority of dietary proteins undergo extensive digestion, small, nutritionally insignificant amounts of food proteins appear to cross the gastrointestinal mucosa intact. Experiments in a variety of allergic models have demonstrated that exposure of the gastrointestinal mucosa to the intact allergen leads to an anaphylactoid reaction. To examine the uptake of immunologically intact protein across the gastrointestinal epithelium, the

mucosal to serosal movement of bovine serum albumin was measured in stripped gastric and intestinal mucosa mounted in modified Ussing-type chambers. Studies demonstrated that both gastric and intestinal mucosa are capable of actively transporting intact dietary proteins. In the intestine, the transport of intact molecules across the epithelium is a saturable, energy dependent process which utilizes the microtubular network and is regulated by the enteric nervous system. Transport across gastric mucosa is also dependent upon the microtubular network and is energy dependent (D.G. Gall, Zhonghua Min Guo Xiao Er Ke Yi Xue Hui Za Zhi, *Gastrointestinal uptake of macromolecules,* 1998 Jan-Feb;39[1]:9 11).

Undigested Maillard molecules suspected to play a role in cancer obviously cross the intestinal barrier. Otherwise, they could never have a carcinogenic, or mutagenic, effect on the body's cells.

Metabolic transit data on food-borne advanced MRPs (Maillard reaction products) termed melanoidins are not yet completely elucidated, and it is still an open question whether isolated melanoidin structures undergo metabolic biotransformation and subsequently cause physiological effects in vivo . . . Advanced MRPs, acting as premelanoidins, and melanoidins are formed under severe heat treatment of foods and are ingested with the habitual diet at considerable amounts. Metabolic transit data are known for Amadori compounds classified as early MRPs, e.g., fructose-lysine. For rats and humans, the percentages of ingested free versus protein-bound fructose-lysine excreted in the urine were found within ranges of 60-80 percent and 3-10 percent, respectively. Balance studies on free advanced MRPs are still lacking, but protein-bound low-molecular-weight premelanoidins and high-molecular weight melanoidins have already been investigated in animal experiments using (14)C-tracer isotopes. The amount of ingested radioactivity absorbed and excreted in the urine was found at levels ranging from 16 to 30 percent and from 1 to 5 percent for premelanoidins and melanoidins, respectively. These different metabolic transit data of premelanoidins and melanoidins can be explained by the following mechanisms involved: (i) intestinal degradation by digestive and microbial enzymes; (ii) absorption of these compounds or their degradates, and (iii) tissue retention. Structure specific in vivo effects have been identified for protein-bound premelanoidins on intestinal microbial activity, xenobiotic biotransformation enzymes and further glycation reactions. The latter are hypothesized to be involved in the aging process and in the course of different diseases. Further investigations are needed to clarify synergistic in vivo effects of dietary ingested melanoidins and endogenously formed glycation products. (V. Faist, H.F. Erbersdobler, *Metabolic Transit and in vivo Effects of Melanoidins*

and Precursor Compounds Deriving from the Maillard Reaction, Ann Nutr
Metab 2001;45[1]:1-12.)

In a perfect world, the immune (or defense) system would identify
incoming molecules (either individually or as part of a larger aggregate)
as useful (to be welcomed) or potentially harmful (to be eliminated).
The unusable material in the food, along with cellular wastes, should
normally be eliminated via the emunctory system. After repeated exposure to those denatured molecules, the immune system enters into a
state of immunological tolerance. The immune system "gives up," in a
sense, and lets abnormal molecules freely enter the body. Such phenomena can be observed when a new smoker may experience dizziness
with the first cigarettes, but over time, as the body enters a state of tolerance, harmful elements contained in the smoke will accumulate in the
lungs and more generally in the body via the bloodstream.

> In summary, synthetic peptides corresponding to linear sequences of HLA class
> I molecules can inhibit T-cell responses in vitro and in vivo. These peptides
> induce immunologic tolerance by binding to hsp-70 family members, causing
> an increase in intracellular calcium, and down-regulating the nuclear factor of
> activated T cells, NF-AT. We suggest that heat shock proteins may function as
> novel immunophilins. Like cyclophilins and FK 506 binding proteins, heat
> shock proteins are ubiquitous, are involved in protein folding and trafficking,
> and bind exogenous drugs. Cyclosporine and FK 506 exert immunosuppres-
> sive effects by binding immunophilins, which as a result interrupt the phos-
> phatase activity of calcineurin. Although the precise pathways involved in the
> synthetic HLA peptide effects are not as well worked out, it seems likely that
> peptide binding to heat shock protein is disrupting normal events in T-cell
> activation, giving rise to an apparently permanent state of anergy (A.M.
> Krensky, C. Clayberger, *Immunologic tolerance: tailored antigen,* Transplant
> Proc 1996 Aug;28[4]:2075-7).

Similarly, early in life, unless a mother was a heavy consumer of dairy
products before her baby was born, when the baby was first given cow's
milk, he probably had some minor diarrhea, vomiting, fever, or rash.
The body's complaints were detoxination attempts, but were not understood by the parents or pediatrician, because milk is considered to be a
natural and wholesome food in our society. The newborn was probably
diagnosed as allergic, and it was expected that the allergy would go away.
And it probably did. After being inescapably subjected to cow's milk for a

week or two, the immunological system began to tolerate it. The human body functions as a whole, inseparable from its environment, and its physiological functions are analogous to its psychological ones: it will tolerate discomforts it can neither flee nor fight.

An immunologic state of tolerance allows unhealthy, toxic, carcinogenic, and mutagenic molecules to build up in cells and organs. Abnormal molecules will be stored in the cellular vacuoles or elsewhere in the cells, or between them, or in special storage (fat) cells. Once past the body's self-defined threshold, the accumulation of unwanted molecules disturbs the organs' vital functions and opens the way to all kinds of pathologies and degenerative diseases.

Advanced glycation end-products (AGEs) are formed by spontaneous chemical reactions between carbohydrates and tissue proteins. The accumulation of AGEs in long-lived proteins contributes to the age-related increase in brown colour, fluorescence and insolubilisation of lens crystallins and to the gradual crosslinking and decrease in elasticity of connective tissue collagens with age. These nonenzymatic reactions, known collectively as Maillard or browning reactions, are also implicated in the development of pathophysiology in age-related diseases such as diabetes mellitus, atherosclerosis, Alzheimer's disease, and in dialysis-related amyloidosis. Oxygen and oxidation reactions accelerates Maillard reactions in vitro, and the structurally characterised AGEs that accumulate in long-lived tissue proteins are in fact glycoxidation products, formed by sequential glycation and oxidation reactions. In addition to their immediate effects on protein structure and function, AGEs also induce oxidative stress, leading to inflammation and propagation of tissue damage. Thus, glycation of protein, formation of AGEs and resultant oxidative stress, which accelerate Maillard reactions, can initiate an autocatalytic cycle of deleterious reactions in tissues. Pharmacological inhibition of the Maillard reaction should improve the prognosis for a broad range of age-related diseases. The role of oxidative stress as a catalyst and the consequences of Maillard reaction damage in tissues suggest that antioxidant therapy may also retard the progression of age-related pathology (S.R. Thorpe, J.W. Baynes, *Role of the Maillard reaction in diabetes mellitus and diseases of aging*, Drugs Aging 1996 Aug;9[2]:69-77).

We do not generally realize how much just a little can do. Very minute amounts of a substance, even in the form of a vapor, may have overwhelming effects on our bodies. A millionth of a gram of chloroform can knock a 150-pound adult unconscious. The ingestion of as little as 1/1,500,000 gram of a botulism toxin can be fatal. Numerous chemicals in undetectable, or barely detectable, amounts can cause blindness, paralysis, or death (and particularly in the case of man-made molecules, they may carry no odor). Homeopathic remedies demonstrate how dramatic effects on the body may be produced by amounts of chemicals so minute that it is impossible even to detect their presence. In fact, in some cases, the fewer there are, the greater their effect. You may find it difficult to realize just how potent "almost nothing" can be. But consider how homeopathic preparations, for example, are typically made by dilutions. One drop of a saturated solution of a chemical agent is mixed with a hundred drops of distilled water in a recipient; then a single drop of this new solution is mixed with a hundred drops of distilled water in another recipient; then one drop of this newly diluted solution is mixed with a hundred times its volume in another recipient, and so on, as many as fifteen times and more. If you will divide one by a hundred, by a hundred, and then again ten or fifteen times, you will begin to see what this means. You might even wish to experiment, starting with one drop of India ink in a hundred drops of water, and see how far you get before the color disappears. By the fifteenth dilution — and in fact, well before — the amount of the original substance appears to be gone, and yet, its effect on the body may often be greater in the higher dilutions than in the lower. So it should not surprise us that even very small numbers of abnormal molecules from our everyday menu, undetectable by laboratory methods (either because there are so few present, or because we do not know what to look for), can produce significant symptoms.

People who have gone through the successive detoxination waves Genefit Nutrition produces know from experience that the amount of abnormal molecules previously accumulated in the body is, for most of us, far from negligible. And yet triggering detoxination with a return to a truly natural diet is the best protection against molecules that can become harmful over time. In the beginning, detoxination waves are triggered every time an immunologic state of tolerance, in relation to a specific class of molecules, is broken by the introduction of a close-kind, unprocessed food. Every time the body enters into contact with a particular unprocessed food, it is like a wake-up call for the immune system, restoring the opportunity to return to the natural order of things. The body is more reactive to some products than others. It all depends on your dietary past and what classes of molecules have been accumulated in your cells. For example, fish seems to be a strong detoxination agent for dairy product molecules. It is not unusual to smell that specific cheese or creamy sauce recipes you ate years ago coming out of your perspiration, urine, and feces after the consumption of tuna fish for example. For people who have passed the first detoxination waves and are on Genefit Nutrition for longer periods of time, the odor of dairy products after consumption of fish will cease eventually, which suggests that those odors do not come from the fish itself.

When the state of tolerance gets disrupted, the immune system suddenly identifies a specific class of molecules as being foreign, and from that point on, the body's waste-management organization takes over. The unwanted molecules are ejected from cells and cellular tissues and enter the bloodstream, before being eliminated by the body through the intestine, perspiration, greasy hair, etc. Once in the bloodstream, those molecules have a similar, immediate effect as they would if you had eaten the processed food they come from. Sometimes the immediate effects are even stronger, because the concentration of harmful molecules can be higher during detoxination than after a cooked meal. That is why it is so important to control the detoxination by carefully controlling the intake quantity of every food. When the intake quantity is not controlled by the nutritional instinct, the detoxination can sometimes be too strong for the body's capacity to handle it. In this case, the detoxination symptoms will include headaches, excessive fatigue, sore muscles, and fever. To avoid this, it is very important to carefully interrogate the nutritional instinct, especially every time a new food is introduced into the palette. It is also beneficial to ease detoxination itself by drinking water, doing exercise, take some fresh air, smell and eat herbs, so the time abnormal molecules spend in the bloodstream and lymph is kept to a minimum.

Experience has shown that for Western people, the unprocessed foods our bodies may be the most reactive to are seafood and meat, probably because of the kinship with the proteins of cooked meat and diary products. This is most likely why these foods have a powerful therapeutic effect on serious pathologies. Tropical fruits, because of our very ancient genetic adaptation to them, are excellent cleansers too. But, in general, no arbitrary rule can be drawn, because detoxination phenomena are always unpredictable. Nevertheless, caution is advised every time one of these foods is introduced; it might save you from unpleasant detoxination episodes.

When controlled by the nutritional instinct, we have never seen a detoxination produce irreversible damage to the body, even if the effects are sometimes spectacular. For example, in some rare cases people get an immunologic reaction on the skin after eating fish: the skin turns fire red within a few minutes after consumption and starts itching. Usually, these symptoms disappear after a couple of hours, or one night of good sleep.

Once the immune system has fully woken up, because the tolerance state has been broken repeatedly, it will be vigorous, alert, extremely discerning and intolerant. It will, among many other things, ensure that not even semi-digested roasted peanut molecules start through the doors of the digestive system. They will be sent packing and be given a chance for so little interaction with the body that they will emerge smelling exactly the way they smelled when they entered. A vigorous immune system will also destroy and eject any intrusive substance, including microbes, amoebas, parasites, splinters, and poisons along with the body's own mutant cells, as soon as they appear. People having vigorous immune systems thanks to Genefit Nutrition are generally immune to infections, and even to neoplasms or tumors.

Under Genefit Nutritional conditions, symptoms coming along with an ejection of abnormal material should be understood to be health restoring. Under so-called "normal" conditions, they will usually be perceived as destructive, something to be "fought," and repressed as quickly as possible. "Normal," denatured diets do, in fact, so exacerbate macroscopic physiological and psychological signs, as a result of the underlying submicroscopic and microscopic chaos they produce, that symptoms may, indeed, easily become unbearable and even potentially lethal. So, it makes sense that in its nonawareness of the profound effects of food, traditional, allopathic medicine should be to treat (eradicate) symptoms. It makes even more sense if the assumption is made, as it generally is, that an absence of patently unpleasant symptoms equals good health. If we define a state of good health as a state of absence of abnormal molecules in the body, then the "normal" population in so-called "good health" is not in good health at all.

We should remember that the science (or art) of medicine is a social calling. It can only be based on the study of sickness and well-being in the society in which it evolved. Its practitioners, as members of that society, share its beliefs. If society at large makes no distinction between genetically natural and unnatural foods, medical practitioners are not likely to either. And historically, no society on record has ever done so. We know of no people on earth, since the advent of agriculture, that have ever had a diet devoid of denatured foods. So, from their very beginnings, until this day, medical theories, research, diagnoses, and treatments have without exception been dealing with populations whose functioning was not truly normal for humans. It has been denatured by abnormal diets. We were never able to recognize this before, because no studies had ever been made of truly well-nourished people, who were eating foods to which they were genetically adapted, in kind and amount determined by their innate biochemical demands. These studies are now under way. They are providing a new frame of reference and new standards for health and disease. And they are radically changing our notions of what "normal" means for human beings. Because they call for a revision of many current assumptions in medicine, nutrition, and other related fields, these studies may not always be welcome.

Most of the unpleasant symptoms we know of have been traditionally perceived in medicine as something to be destroyed by executing the "agent" that "caused" them. One reason for this is that medicine has been ignorant (as we all have) of the toxins in denatured food. Not realizing they were there, we could not understand their effects. But it is now clear that food is a major causative factor in most, if not all, illnesses. This includes even some conditions not usually thought of as abnormal at all. And it is clear that whatever the symptoms, their severity directly reflects the degree of intoxination. In other words, the fewer the nutritional toxins in the body, the fewer and/or milder the symptoms, regardless of any viral, microbial, or other pathogenic agents that may be present. When nutritional toxins are at a level that is truly normal for humans, humans become:

1. immune to inflammatory pain,
2. immune to infections, and
3. free of abnormal odors.

These phenomena occur very rarely in people eating the usual "balanced" diets of processed foods, and almost universally in people eating unprocessed foods selected by instinct. Although individuals with an extremely high level of intoxination may also seem free of symptoms as usually defined, they nevertheless remain subject to infections and pain, and continue to carry body odors.

There is a fundamental difference between symptoms produced when nutritional toxins are leaving the body and symptoms occurring because they have not. By analogy, if you clean your house by sweeping the dirt out the door, you will raise a lot of dust, but the house will be left clean, and you can repeat the process when needed. On the other hand, if your method is to sweep the dirt under the rug, sooner or later, the place will become too dirty to live in, no matter how often you sweep it. If you were standing down the street watching the first kind of house cleaning, you might see, along with the dust clouds, dog hair, food scraps, bits of a broken glass, and a torn shoelace emerging through doors and windows. You might even see an old chair or TV set tossed out. A similar situation holds for the human body. Nutritional toxins, like dust, may emerge at any one of the body's numerous "doors" or "windows" into the outside world — in other words, at every point where body cells are in touch with the environment.

Although we usually think of the skin as the "outside" of our bodies, we do in fact also touch our environment through the mouth, ears, lungs, sinuses, stomach, intestines, vagina, and elsewhere. At a cellular level, the interface between the inside and the outside of an adult human being is enormous. The total contact surface of an adult's intestines covers about 2,700 square feet — the size of a tennis court. If each cell were scaled to the size of a Coke bottle, the area covered would be larger than Manhattan. The lungs, with all their substructures, would cover an entire city as well.

Normally, the body does not eliminate wastes at equal rates over its entire "surface," but uses specific channels: primarily the bladder, intestines, and bowels, and secondarily, the skin and lungs. Normal elimination of the body's natural waste happens spontaneously and passes almost unnoticed. It is a natural function, and its mechanisms are inherent to us, the genetically determined product of millions of years of natural evolution. But our normal cleansing capacity is also a product of evolution, and this is where problems arise in today's industrialized environment. When we are required to process and discharge types and amounts of toxins going far beyond those found in nature, our normal processes become overtaxed, or may no longer suffice at all. Then, abnormal (nonusual) processes are forced into play. And these, when they become severe enough to be noticed, are what we call "symptoms." When do symptoms indicate that toxins are leaving the body? If we can identify these symptoms, perhaps we can also have enough good sense to avoid thwarting the beneficial cleansing.

The Symptoms of Detoxination

1. There is a discharge of bodily matter carrying abnormal odors. The matter may be fluid, in the form of pus, sputum, or vaginal discharge, or it may be seemingly dry, in the form of dandruff, a rash, or flaking skin. If the only matter being discharged is the normally occurring urine and feces, detoxination is signified by the presence of abnormal odors. Symptoms that are signs of detoxination are useful for the body, even if sometimes temporarily unpleasant. If they are unusual, it is because they constitute unusual methods of cleaning, needed when the ordinary methods are not "up to the job." Always remember, the more rarely you bring muddy boots into the house, the less intensely it will have to be cleaned.

2. The symptoms are spontaneously self-terminating. They will spontaneously disappear once no nutritional toxins of that given class are left to be flushed out. The kinds of symptoms known to be spontaneously self-terminating are, in fact, cleansing processes. Do not shut doors and windows while house cleaning is in progress! It is extremely important for the long-term integrity of the organism that detoxination symptoms are allowed to occur unmolested. Suppressing them with drugs may seemingly "cure" them in the short run, but the drugs will cause toxins

to accumulate further in the body. Unless they are so severe as to endanger life or produce irreversible damage, no prescription is necessary for detoxination symptoms other than raw, unprocessed food and fresh water. Limiting intervention to these elements alone will, in most cases, spontaneously cause the symptoms to subside in short order.

3. There is fever in conjunction with the two preceding criteria. When fever occurs, it means blood circulation throughout the body's tissues has increased dramatically because the organism called for it. In other words, the body needs the increased irrigation. Fever is a system-wide phenomenon. Where fever occurs in association with at least one of the first two criteria, it is a toxin-related symptom and it is recommended not to suppress it, unless it is unbearable or represents a danger to life. An effort should be made to ease or lower detoxination by paying close attention to the nutritional instinct's signals and drinking enough water. Fever that is not obviously associated with detoxination should, of course, be evaluated and treated medically (as should any other symptoms) with this proviso.

If you actually use the method of Genefit Nutrition, you will soon be able to recognize detoxination symptoms when they occur. If you avoid intoxinating yourself further at that time, you will prevent the symptoms from becoming severe and hasten their disappearance. And if you can avoid reverting to a high-toxicity diet, you will soon find yourself in better health than you ever thought possible.

Under conditions of Genefit Nutrition, it is even common for a person to be relieved of prior complaints to which the illness was apparently unrelated. A multiple sclerosis patient will be delighted when he catches a cold (a typical detoxination illness), because it promises an improvement in his condition. It is obvious from his odors that his sputum, sweat, urine, and feces are carrying with it abnormal molecules that had accumulated in his body. We would not detect them under normal nutritional conditions, because normally the person would still be ingesting denatured soups, juices, tea, and other cooked foods, whose odors would also be present. It may seem unusual to suggest some illnesses, including contagious diseases, such as influenza and hepatitis, could be salutary for a person's long-term well being. But under strict Genefit eating conditions, it is clear they have that effect. For those suffering from autoimmune or neoplastic pathology, or other diseases of civilization, it is doubly important that detoxination symptoms be allowed to run their course without being suppressed. By enabling the body to redirect energies from garbage detail to construction crew, these symptoms are invaluable aids to self-healing.

Observation brought us to infer that microbes or other agents associated with an illness are not necessarily its *cause*. Even where particular sets of symptoms are associated with specific types of microorganisms, it does not mean they happened *because* of them. No symptoms would appear if the conditions that allow them to appear weren't present; infectious agents alone are not enough. Naive cause and effect reasoning has a blinding effect, even upon physicians who recognize the multiple factors underlying pathology. Pasteur, who discovered microbes in the first place, advised his peers they carried less responsibility for disease than the state of the body itself. But his words have too often gone unheeded.

The associated "pathogenic" microorganisms may, in fact, be feeding upon accumulated nutritional toxins the body would be unable to eliminate without assistance. Remember, without bacterial help, we would be unable to process even natural food and its wastes in the first place: we carry a greater number of bacteria in our intestinal tracts than cells in our bodies, many of which are vital to digestion.

All living organisms are subject to the laws of the survival of the fittest, and infectious microorganisms are no exception. Like other living beings, they mutate and evolve in response to their environments, food sources included. This is how strains of bacteria have emerged that are not only resistant to penicillin or other antibiotics, but actually thrive on them. So, it is not far-fetched at all to infer some microbes may actually be rendering us a service via their ability to thrive upon abnormal molecules we would be unable to eliminate without their help.

> If a comparison is made between a slice of meat from a steer fed exclusively on grass in a pasture, and free from vaccines and artificially injected hormones, and meat from a steer that ate hay, grains, or industrial fodders, it is found that the commercially raised meat begins to turn — begins to harbor a large bacterial population — within two or three days while meat from the animal fed original food will not turn for two to three weeks. (Schutte & Meyers, *Metabolic Aspects of Health*, Discovery Press, Kentfield, CA, 1979.)

We might even wonder whether a majority of the extraneous microbes found in the world today are better adapted genetically to pollutants than to the absence of pollutants. This might partially explain why people on Genefit are immune to infections in cuts and bruises (immuno-logical defenses notwithstanding): perhaps microbes that are adapted to denatured food toxins can find little or nothing to thrive on in their absence! And it reflects the fact that someone on Genefit Nutrition can still become ill with a detoxination "illness" (generally in a benign form) if he has not previously eliminated abnormal molecules that the agents of the illness are, in fact, feeding upon (thus breaking those agents down, making their elimination possible).

There are no such things as good guys and bad guys in the natural world, only organisms, which are trying to survive. If humans harbor diseases, there is a reason for them that has nothing to do with evil intent on the part of microscopic "invaders": no creature, except man, tries to hurt another, except in order to eat, reproduce, or defend itself. If the microorganisms to which we fall prey were not somehow pertinent to our integrity, we would never have evolved so as to attract them to us. Even millions of years ago, there would have been some ingestion of accidentally denatured foods and extraneous material the body could not metabolize or eliminate properly without special help. Fast-mutating germs on the lookout for a meal, and able to quickly adapt to a novel one, would have filled the bill. Under instinctive eating conditions, alien microorganisms entering our bodies are either always kept well in check or destroyed by our immune systems, if dangerous to the body's integrity. Only when the immune system is not working properly can their population explode and produce acute symptoms.

Of course, this is not in line with medical thinking based on Aristotle, Newton, and Euclid. But in today's world, a thing can both "be" and "not be," matter is no longer "solid," and lines are no longer "straight." It is time medicine was brought up to date. If it has not yet happened, one of the reasons is, not logic, but food. Mind is not separate from body. From the ends of our toes to the tips of our tongues, we are what we eat — ideas and feelings, perceptions and dreams included.

NOTES

1. Schulte & Meyers, *Metabolic Aspects of Health,* Discovery Press, Kentfield CA, 1979.

PART THREE

Do It Yourself

ELEVEN

Before You Jump

AFTER YOU HAVE READ and understood the theoretical aspects of Genefit Nutrition you will probably wonder how you can apply it in your life. The following chapters will give you practical guidelines for a successful jump.

Even if the principles of Genefit Nutrition appear to be simple, their application in most cases is not, as there are many hindering physiological and psychological factors involved.

If you should decide to apply Genefit Nutrition for more than three days we strongly recommend you consult our Online Tutorial or order our CD-ROM. Even if guidelines in this book address all the most basic practical aspects, more extensive knowledge will noticeably increase you chances of success. If you should encounter insurmountable difficulties in your practice, don't get the results you have expected, or struggle with prolonged detoxination symptoms, we recommend you contact us. Together we will fix the problem.

If you are subject to serious health conditions, supervision is highly recommended. Serious pathological conditions need special care, and guidelines in this book may not suffice. Here again contact us and together we will find the best way to proceed.

Now, let's get ready.

First of all, several application options are available to you:

- If you are not quite sure yet if Genefit Nutrition is for you, you might simply want to give it a try. We recommend a quick cleansing program of three days. With a three-day program you won't have to face the psychological challenges that come along when you practice for longer periods yet you will still have a first insight of what Genefit Nutrition is all about.

- If you are ready for the big jump we recommend you limit yourself to twenty-one days for the first time.

WHY TWENTY-ONE DAYS?

Limiting your adventure in time will make it easier on you. You will experience fewer psychological tensions if you know that you can go back to a more traditional diet soon.

When starting to eat instinctively, you will go through different phases.

First, as you implement the principles of Genefit Nutrition, you will experience a three-day transition period while your body physiologically and psychologically adjusts to the new way of eating and gets rid of residues of cooked food from your intestinal tract. Depending on your dietary history, those three days can be more or less challenging.

Don't underestimate the value of movement, water, and rest. Ignoring them slows down detoxination, resulting in uncomfortable symptoms. At this point, you will either give up and go back to the way you were eating, or you may continue, using the principles more fully.

By the second week you will start to notice improvements in your physical, mental, emotional, and creative well-being. You may still be experiencing detoxination phenomena, as detoxination becomes more profound, but this time, they happen more in waves throughout the day, typically towards the end of the morning or around four or five in the afternoon. However, the improved well-being you are experiencing will help you to get through these detoxination waves and will encourage you to continue on your Genefit Nutrition cleanse.

By the third week, you should have experienced how good it is possible to feel. You will have periods of noticeable mental clarity, high levels of energy and physical well-being. This is the particular state we want you to experience; it will serve you as a reference of health for the rest of your life.

With any new endeavor, for maximum success and reward, it is a good idea to prepare yourself. Success is like a formula: leave a bit out and you create a "maybe," maybe it's working, maybe it's not; maybe it works for everyone else but me. Do each step of the formula and the result is guaranteed. Here are some key points for maximum success when you take the step to eat instinctively:

1. Know why Genefit Nutrition works. Everyone from your family and friends to complete strangers will question you about it! Make sure it is your own decision based on knowledge and logic. Your own certainty and understanding is your greatest asset in successfully undertaking this or any new thing.

2. Set a time goal: three or twenty-one days? Some people find it quite natural to continue eating instinctively after those periods. Others use it as a tool in their lives to help when they become run-down, overweight, or just need a "spring cleanse." Everyone will come to their own decision of how they want to utilize Genefit Nutrition.

    During whatever time you set to eat instinctively, be aware, you will initially have all kinds of thoughts about what you will eat the day you finish! This can be, for instance, chocolate, ice cream, or simply your favorite meal. However, it is a good idea to wait until you get to the end of your goal to decide, so that cravings and compulsions don't influence your decision.

    After twenty-one days, a noticeably high feeling of well-being will be the indication you are on the right path. Whether you extend your goal or not should depend on whether you have reached this level of "feeling great" within that time.

3. Prepare your family, friends, and work associates. We suggest you keep words like "never again" and "forever" out of your vocabulary. Other people will be able to cope better with the idea of you doing something new if it is for a limited time. Genefit Nutrition is not a part of most people's way of thinking, so when you do tell others, be prepared for their responses. Common responses are usually opposition or interest. Opposition is a challenge in any new endeavor.

Opposition to eating instinctively can range from intense emotional attacks to attempts to get you to have a cigarette or just a little piece of chocolate.

A good strategy can be to avoid the trap of defending yourself. An interested response will usually see you answering lots of questions and testing your knowledge. A determined decision should be enough to enable you to hold your own in any situation and can be kept strong by frequently reviewing your goals.

4. Let yourself be a demonstration of positive improvement, not just a vocal exponent. Take it easy on arrogance. It is easy to fall into the trap of having all the answers. It can be humbling to know that we can always learn something from another, no matter who they are, what they do, or what condition they are in. A know-it-all attitude prevents the acquisition of new knowledge.

5. Prepare your environment, especially the kitchen. Remove all temptations, including cookies, candies, and those "treats" in the freezer. Ideally, get rid of all processed foods.

6. Start eating instinctively one hundred percent. Eating altered foods while eating instinctively causes frustration, dissatisfaction, instinctual confusion, and erratic emotions. It can also make you sick.

7. Watch the quality of the food. The difference between having a strictly unprocessed food supply and having a single processed food in your palette is also the difference between success and failure. One processed food in your choice is enough to jeopardize your practice.

There can be a big difference between good quality, organically grown food and food grown or treated with chemicals. Even if organic is sometimes not enough, it is always preferred. Food grown with chemical fertilizers and pesticides can be altered so that the instinct does not work. This may be the case if you can eat a lot of something without an instinctive stop and then you experience digestive problems.

To solve the food supply problem, research your area. Inform yourself. Where will you buy your food? Which stores and farmers supply fresh, quality food? Which stores and farmers supply organic food? Find out about your local farmers markets. Or, you can also order our 21-day package at The Purefood Network, which contains all the high-quality food you need for a successful ride. We have designed the 21-day package especially for people who don't have easy access to unprocessed food or simply don't have the time to look for it. Either way, our 21-day package will solve the issue. For more information about ordering Purefood, please see page ___.

8. Be sure you have a sufficient variety of foods. If nothing is particularly attractive and a sensation of frustration results, find out if any food is missing. Depending on budget and availability, a course might contain from five to twenty-five different foods belonging to a particular group of foods. The greater the variety, the greater the chance you may discover an item that fills urgent metabolic needs. For a person in fairly good health who is applying Genefit Nutrition for twenty-one days, a more limited selection will probably suffice, but for someone critically ill, the larger the choice, the better the chances of finding foods that will enable him or her to recover.

   If you choose to acquire food by yourself, go to markets and smell your way around! Be careful not to choose mentally your old favorites and automatically reject your past dislikes. As your body's condition changes so will your food preferences.

9. Try Genefit as a group. Gather a bunch of friends and jump into the adventure together. It is much more fun and builds a great environment for mutual support.

10. Study the content of our Online Tutorial or multimedia CD-ROM. It will drastically increase your chances of success.

11. If you are not sure you can do it by yourself, contact us. A certified Genefit Nutrition coach has expertise in getting you through the initial period of eating instinctively. Also, you may want to do our Genefit Nutrition retreat to get started.

Jump Time!

Imagine you have just completed your training to do a parachute jump. Your instructor has given you the training in how to jump, count, position your body in the air, pull the cords, and land. Performing each one is a part of the complete formula for success. Is there any part of that formula that you would leave out? Probably not — because you don't just want to make it to the ground, you want to enjoy every minute of your experience. This and the following chapters are all parts of the success formula for Genefit Nutrition.

TWELVE

Welcome to the Guidelines of Genefit Nutrition

AS WITH ANY NEW DATA, the guidelines of eating instinctively may seem complex or overregulated at first. Once put in practice, however, they correspond simply to the function of the instinct as observed in a healthy body instead of being hard and fast rules. The following is a description of a typical Genefit Nutrition day. It will give you an idea how to structure your meals and your day in general. Take the method described and multiply it by the number of days you decided to apply Genefit Nutrition. Even if the method stays the same, your instinct will make every day a brand new day.

1. In the Morning

First thing in the morning, taste a variety of waters. We recommend avoiding mineral-added waters and tap water, especially if you live in a big city. Several varieties of pure or spring waters will be best. Taste will guide you, just as with food, to the right water. Continue to choose and drink water in the same way throughout the morning, afternoon, and evening. Avoid interfering with digestion by not drinking at, or too soon after, mealtimes. One hour after eating is generally best. Because of the detoxination Genefit Nutrition triggers, you should drink a lot of water throughout the day, relying on taste rather than waiting for thirst.

As an aid to elimination, we recommend taking cassia fistula in the morning and before going to sleep (see Chapter 13).

Many of us have been told we must eat breakfast or we won't have the energy to get through the morning. This may be true for a person on a processed food diet. However, it is more often the reason for a lot of overloaded, toneless, and troubled digestive organs. When eating instinctively it is important not to eat in the morning. Morning is the main detoxifying time for the body, so to eat at this time is cutting off the detoxination process. The body cannot efficiently digest new material and detoxify old molecules at the same time. All signs of discomfort in the morning related to this detoxination process should disappear by the end of first week at the latest, if Genefit Nutrition is applied correctly. In the morning, it is essential to ease the detoxination process, and so see potential symptoms disappear, instead of interrupting it by eating.

2. Have Your First Meal around 12 o'clock

First, drink water before the meal and so avoid looking for fluids instead of nutrients in fruits. Fruit sugars provide the energy needed for daily activity, so it is best to choose from fruits and sweet foods for lunch. (See Chapter 15 for the composition of the 12 o'clock meal.)

Smell all the foods available one after the other. It is important to give them all a chance. In order to avoid past prejudice or automatic habits, do a first round, and only keep the ones that smell pleasant. Eliminate all the others. By now, you should only have a few left. Take them two by two and compare their smells. If you are not sure which one to keep, compare the smell until one will yield to the other. Do this with all remaining foods and proceed by elimination until there is only one left. This is the one your body wants the most. It may be beneficial to close your eyes or use a blindfold when choosing. Have a friend hold each fruit for you to smell without looking at them. In doing so you will not be influence by your mind. The results are often surprising. You may find yourself choosing foods you have avoided for years. Perhaps you had an unpleasant memory or experience of that food, but meanwhile your body needs the nutrients it contains. Or, you may have previously disliked many raw foods because of the toxic condition of your body systems. This is a phenomenon of a processed food diet. Interest, satisfaction, and pleasure in raw foods will increase as the body eliminates the waste from years of storage.

Salivary response is also an important sign of what the body wants and, more specifically, what it is able to metabolize. A pleasant smell should be accompanied by the presence of a salivation reflex. No saliva can mean the body is presently unable to digest the food. Even without the salivary response the food may smell pleasant. In this case, you will have to test this food again at later meals, or perhaps you just need to inhale the aroma without ingesting the food. This can often be the case with herbs.

If the odor of a food is not perceptible, you may need to make a scratch or cut in the surface, heat it with your breath, or in exceptional cases, taste without swallowing.

The main function of the sense of smell is to select food, but smelling also puts you in chemical and energetic tune with the food. Eating randomly will not give you the same level of satisfaction and eating pleasure. The more precisely you choose by smell, the better results you will get.

In this way, choose the food, which is the most attractive and begin to eat it. Continue eating that food until your body gives you an "instinctive stop." Be careful not to just go automatically from one food to another. As long as the chosen food tastes delicious, or until there is an alliesthesial response, continue to eat it. For example, it is not uncommon to see people eating five or six bananas in a row before the body sends out a signal to stop.

Normally, the body will not want more of a food for which there has already been a stop. In other words, once you have had a stop with a particular food, don't go back to it. If you are not satisfied, choose a different food using the same method. It is perfectly normal to choose from one to five different types of food at a lunch meal.

Sometimes it can be quite a change in routine to leave something we have started eating. This is what we have been told not to do since childhood, often under duress: "Clean your plate!" However, it is better to leave the remainder of a food than overload your body with something it cannot use. We are not advocating thoughtless waste, and in fact there is very little waste, especially if those you live with eat instinctively too. The

food that you have had an instinctive stop on may be delicious to someone else.

Most of the time carbohydrate-rich foods will be all you will need at
the midday meal. However, after you have eaten fruits, dates, or honey,
and no other carbohydrate-rich food smells attractive and you still feel
unsatisfied, try herbs or vegetables, selecting by smell, determining the
quantity by taste or other body signals.

Don't be concerned if, at a meal, nothing seems attractive. If no food
smells attractive or stimulates salivation, your body may be detoxifying
and need a salutary fast. If that is the case it is especially important to stay
well hydrated with water. If you have no attraction towards foods for several meals it is an alarm bell indicating that your body is having trouble
eliminating. You should pay particular attention to helping the processes
of elimination (see Chapter 13). You may also need to check that the
quality and variety of your food is good.

3. In the Afternoon

Do not snack in the afternoon! Digestion is a preset program. If you eat
in the afternoon two programs will overlap. The result is digestive discomforts and the loss of the ecstatic phases at the next meal. Smelling
herbs or any other tool from the Toolbox (Chapter 13) is welcome if
detoxination gets too strong.

4. Have Your Evening Meal around 6 or 7 o'clock

Dinner is divided into two main parts:

Proteins and fats: In the first course of the evening meal we include
high-fat and high-protein foods. (See Chapter 15 for the composition of
the 6 o'clock meal.)

Whereas fruits generally supply energy, protein foods are for construction and regeneration. Proteins and fats are more complex to digest so it
is ideal to eat them in the evening. Combining different foods from this
category in a meal creates problems for the digestive and immune sys-

tems. Therefore, it is recommended to choose only one high-fat or high-protein food in the evening meal. Durian, for instance, is a fruit, but contains more protein than many red meats, so it should be included in this category.

Here again drink plenty of water first, so you won't try to satisfy your thirst by choosing juicy foods. Begin your evening meal by choosing the protein or fat food that smells the most attractive and stimulates salivation. Use the same method as at lunch. Eat the chosen food until you get a stop and then go on to vegetables.

It is not mandatory to eat a high-protein or high-fat food every day. During different phases your body might or might not need them. Let your nose guide you. If none of them smell pleasant, go straight to vegetables.

Vegetables: After the high-protein or high-fat food, choose vegetables one at a time, using the same techniques of smell, taste, and awareness of instinctive stops. Eat each chosen food until the taste becomes fairly unpleasant.

It is recommended to choose at least two to six different vegetable sequences in an evening meal.

After the vegetables, if you don't feel satisfied and have had no animal products, smell the fruits.

Do not go more than a day without eating vegetables. This may be a sign that your body needs help with elimination or that the quality, combination, or variety of the foods is not good. It is not recommended to eat a food rich in carbohydrates in combination with an animal protein food. Nor is it recommended to regularly eat a sugar or fruit food with a plant protein or fat food. Eating fruits in the evening should be an exception rather than the rule.

5. At Nighttime

This is the time the body's waste-management system takes over. After the digestion of the evening meal is completed, the detoxination process starts and will extend to the first meal of the next day. This time is important and whatever happens, do not eat. In the evening, even if you don't feel thirsty, test the water if it is attractive to taste. Take cassia as in the morning to ease the detoxination process during the night.

6. Recognizing the Instinctive Signals

The general rule is: *The more pleasure we have with a food's smell and taste, the more it matches our body's needs.*

This is not true for denatured foods artificially made so attractive that we need to limit consumption by using our mind.

As you eat instinctively you will become more experienced at recognizing the instinctive signals. You now know that an instinctive stop is the body signaling that it either doesn't need or has had enough of a food. Initially, one may think that one isn't getting instinctive stops, but usually it is just a matter of recognizing them. This is where a real-life seminar, a Genefit Nutrition retreat, or our one-on-one coaching services can help. One of the advantages of beginning with a Genefit Nutrition coach or a retreat group is that you are immediately hearing about, observing, and experiencing different kinds of stops.

Some of the changes in your body indicating an instinctive stop are:

- *Taste:* from sweet or pleasant to bitter, tasteless, too sweet, or too salty
- *Saliva:* from "mouth-watering" to a drying-up or an absence of saliva, feeling thirsty
- *Flavor:* from pleasant or delicious to unpleasant or no flavor
- *Texture:* from moist to doughy or pasty
- *Comfort:* from comfortable to full, hot, flushed, hiccups, burping, cramps, pain, or burning
- *Fullness:* from not feeling your stomach at all to a sensation of volume or fullness.

Another sign from the body that it does not want a food, or has had enough, is the sensation of disgust ("dis" = against, "gust" = taste). Disgust can mean that a food would bring on too strong a detoxination if eaten.

There are as many different instinctive stops as there are different body conditions. From these examples, you can see that an instinctive stop may not only manifest as change in smell or taste, but that it can be any kind of body response. Gustatory and olfactory alliesthesia is pure instinct and acts as an exclusive guide in people and animals with a non-intoxicated body. Other instinctive stops are in direct connection with the regulation of detoxination and occur because of the presence of abnormal molecules that have to be eliminated.

Salads are raw, but because they are mixtures, the senses cannot tell which of the ingredients are needed and which are not. Munching on apples "when you feel like it" or downing raw steaks is not the way to use the instinct. If a person wants results he needs to apply Genefit Nutrition correctly. With Genefit Nutrition, the key to optimal nutrition is pleasure. Pleasure is the immediate reward for listening to your body. Many people will have to learn to accept it without guilt. With denatured foods, pleasure often leads to trouble. We may enjoy ice cream, chocolates, buttered popcorn, and soft drinks, and almost inevitably pay a price: nausea, indigestion, a hangover, hives, and so on — not to mention the heartburn for which so many pharmaceutical remedies are currently formulated in America. As a consequence, in our "normal" nutritional universe, we come to believe that what is pleasurable isn't good for us, and that for something to be good for us, it must not be pleasurable.

With unprocessed foods, just the opposite is true. In nature, what an animal wants is one and the same as what it needs. This applies to humans also. If someone does not enjoy a food, he will not want it, and he shouldn't eat it because if he doesn't enjoy it, he doesn't need it.

For the first few days, most people do not enjoy unprocessed food as much as food that is cooked and seasoned. Their senses of smell and taste are still dull partially as a result of overloads. They are also desensitized by the abnormal molecules still in the body, which came from the processed foods eaten previously. Until these unnatural materials are cleaned out, the senses remain denatured too. They will progressively become much more acute, and along with them, eyesight, intuition, and hearing. Thinking generally becomes clearer too. But all this will not happen overnight, and the newcomer will need to be patient and persevere. Once you get the hang of Genefit Nutrition, it becomes second nature. After all, it was already with us when we were born. Within a short time, you will notice that the taste of a food varies with practically every bite. It will feel alive.

Within two or three weeks, if you are making no dietary transgressions, you will probably be enjoying original foods more than denatured ones.

If, from the beginning, you make no exceptions to eating unprocessed foods exclusively selected by smell and taste (not by thinking), it will become fairly easy to eat regularly this way with ever-increasing pleasure. Once your senses have opened up, you may experience extraordinary pleasure with food the body needs. However, dietary transgressions — "Oh, just one little candy bar won't hurt" — will have the effect of desensitizing the palate. When the next meal is less satisfying, temptation is increased to have another snack on the side, which in turn will cause less enjoyment at the next meal, and so on in a vicious circle. Once you start making dietary exceptions, you may quickly find yourself back where you started.

7. Need or Deception

If you do not have a stop with a food, most of the time it will be because your body still needs it. In this case, there is also an associated feeling of well-being and an absence of digestive symptoms afterwards. Conversely, if you experience symptoms and discomforts after consumption, there may be no instinctive stop because the food has been processed. If this happens, immediately eliminate this food from your choice, as keeping it will prevent you from enjoying the benefits Genefit Nutrition has to offer.

8. Food Combining

When you begin to eat instinctively after a diet of processed foods, it is like recalibrating your mind to listen to the instinct. After a while, especially when you have detoxified your body, using the instinct to eat will seem more natural than being guided by rules. Initially, the evidence of a poor food combination can often be found in the aftereffects, e.g., bloating and flatulence. The combination to avoid, which by experience and observation seems to hold true most of the time, is that of proteins (especially animal proteins) and carbohydrate-rich or sweet foods. Instinct, pleasure, satisfaction, and no digestive problems are the best guidelines of all.

You will soon come to recognize your body's language and have certainty about your progress. Some questions to continue to consider are: During and after eating, is there symptom-free digestion? You should not experience problems such as gas, uncomfortable fullness, pain, burping, and heartburn! Are there feelings of satisfaction, lightness, clarity, or pleasant aftertaste? The proof that the instinct is being followed and combinations of foods are good will ultimately be found in the sensations and feelings of perfect digestion and well-being.

THIRTEEN

The Other Half of Success —
Your Toolbox

MOST OF US used to a diet of cooked, processed foods have sluggish, under-performing body systems. Your body will probably need some help to get moving! Eating unprocessed food instinctively is the first step. Getting the waste out of your body is the other, equally important step. To do the first and not the second is heading for trouble. From the very first day, detoxination phenomena will appear. The faster and more efficiently the body is able to eliminate, the less discomfort will be experienced physically, emotionally, and mentally. It is when the waste is accumulated in the bloodstream, lymph, bowels, muscles, and joints that you will experience discomfort.

Eating instinctively will dislodge toxins from the cells. The following list of tools will help complete the toxins' journey out of the body. Besides cassia, you will not need to use all of them every day. You will come to know your body very well and will intuitively know which tools to reach for. You doubtless will also find your own tools as you relearn your own body. Here are nine tried-and-true tools to ensure your detoxination to be as effective and comfortable as possible:

TOOL #1: CASSIA

Cassia fistula is a tree from the cassia family. This naturally occurring gourd grows wild in tropical climates such as southern Mexico, Thailand,

Indonesia, and Hawaii. This fruit was used as a natural laxative in Europe at the beginning of the twentieth century. It looks like a hand-rolled cigar about two feet long. The gourd contains compartments with seeds in them, separated by small disks coated with a black, licorice-like substance that can smell delicious or rotten depending on need. The disks are sucked until the taste begins to bite the tongue and throat. Cassia is a blood purifier and a purgative. It acts by stimulating the elimination of toxins from the cells to the blood and from the blood to the intestines. As such it is a powerful and effective aid when detoxifying. Without it the detoxination will be slower and more difficult, with an increase in secretions from the skin, and mucus from the lungs and sinuses. Cassia is such an effective cleanser that it is mandatory for any successful Genefit Nutrition cleanse and should be regularly used by anyone who is making a serious effort to recover his health through Genefit Nutrition.

Finding the right dose and giving your body a chance to take advantage of it progressively is important. Too much will bring on too strong a detoxination, which can cause digestive discomforts. In order to prevent this, begin with five pieces of cassia and double every day until you reach a stop. The instinctive stop with cassia is usually a burning in the mouth, but other stops can also occur. It may provoke diarrhea at first, which later becomes infrequent. If diarrhea is too frequent or if there is slight abdominal pain, it is best to cut the amount in half the next day rather than omit the cassia altogether. If no further discomfort appears, double the dose again the next day. The amount of old, stored waste that can be eliminated as feces when taking cassia can be quite incredible. It is obvious that it is waste because of the distinctive smells.

If, after two to three weeks of taking cassia, there are still occasions of diarrhea, it is probably not due to the cassia, but some highly concentrated toxins the body needs to get rid of as fast as possible. Diarrhea is one way the body uses to accelerate cleansing. Again, if this happens, it is best not to stop taking cassia, but listen to your sense of taste to regulate the intake.

Cassia is best taken in the morning or before going to sleep, after one is well hydrated with water, but it is not recommended to drink water right after taking cassia. However, cassia can also be taken in the afternoon if the body needs extra help with elimination. If you experience detox discomforts, eat a small amount at least an hour before the evening meal.

It is not recommended to take large amounts of cassia if you are not eating a hundred percent instinctively. The effect will be confusion for your body and the creation of an overly strong detoxination. Cassia is not always easily available in nontropical countries. If you can't find it easily, contact the The Purefood Network.

TOOL # 2: DRINK!

Keep your body well hydrated. All the work of dislodging and eliminating waste requires a fluid medium, so don't wait until you are thirsty to drink water. People can drink large amounts of water while detoxifying (one gallon or more a day in exceptional cases). As long as water runs down your throat easily, drink it. Also remember there are many kinds of water, so try different ones, choosing what is most attractive. Water is the only beverage for Genefit practitioners, because others have been denatured. Every cell exists in and contains a medium of fluid. Drinking enough water will help ensure that the processes of elimination of waste from the cells goes smoothly and comfortably.

TOOL # 3: MOVE!

Movement is vital, especially in the first few weeks of eating instinctively. Movement is like self-massage, inside and out.

By moving we are not just toning up muscles and organs but also stimulating the lymphatic system, which is similar in structure to our vascular system and looks like a complex road map. Lymph conveys nutrients and carries out waste products. In other words, it delivers the good stuff and picks up the garbage. The lymph capillaries and vessels have many valves, which create a "one-way street" system, preventing backflow. To make room for fresh lymph, and to help keep moving the garbage collection along, there needs to be muscle contractions and body and limb movement. So, while the vascular system has the heart as a pump to keep it circulating, the lymphatic system needs movement to keep it going and prevent stagnation of waste. Feeling ill can be a direct result of the garbage not being collected and dumped.

In our experience, those who get their body moving with some form of exercise every day experience a markedly more comfortable, often symptom-free, detoxination. Exercise is especially important in the morning, which is usually the most intense detoxination time. Walking (starting with about thirty minutes and increasing up to at least an hour), dancing, rollerblading, swimming, yoga, and gentle rebounding (mini-trampoline) are some examples of exercise that will greatly assist you. Choose what you enjoy! We recommend that your choice of exercise not be too strenuous or "violent" so as not to interfere with the body's pace of detoxination.

It is an unfortunate fact, proven by most of us who have been through the initial detoxination, that when you least feel like doing anything — you have a headache, no energy, feel sleepy or grumpy — it is because of what is hanging around inside your body waiting to be eliminated. Of course this is the time to get yourself up and moving. Just do it! It becomes easier and easier as you get results, especially when a headache or "cold" symptoms disappear five minutes into a walk. If you sit around, the waste will also sit around.

TOOL # 4: BREATHE!

Breathing is essential for life. Make your breathing quality breathing by really filling up your lungs and exhaling fully. Three big breaths like that in the morning, when you're walking or when your elimination feels sluggish, can really get things moving. Your body will appreciate the extra oxygen, your circulation will improve, your lungs will eliminate waste with each exhalation, and your skin will look alive and healthy. Quality breathing is a priceless tool — and it's free!

TOOL # 5: SKIN BRUSHING

Use a dry loufah sponge on your skin before a shower or walk. Move in circular, sweeping motions up from your feet and then from your fingers towards your body while holding your arm above your heart. This move-ment towards your heart helps stimulate blood and lymph flow, thereby helping your skin, the largest organ of the body, to eliminate dead cells and waste. Even used while showering, a loufah sponge is a natural, inexpensive way to exfoliate.

TOOL # 6: MASSAGE

Massage can be relaxing and enjoyable. It is also an effective way of stimulating circulation of blood and lymph, which is why people sometimes get a headache or muscle pain after a massage because it has stirred up some toxins. Drink water before and after your massage and, if there are any discomforts, go for a walk and/or breathe deeply until they are gone.

While eating instinctively and detoxifying it is preferable to have gentle massage only. We also recommend that you don't have deep-tissue massage while detoxifying so as not to interfere with your body's own pace of detoxination. If any, we suggest very mild saunas and steam room sessions for the same reason.

TOOL # 7: TAKE A BATH!

A warm bath can give your body that extra help it needs to eliminate toxins. Don't be surprised if you end up with discolored bath water. It isn't very pleasant but it means waste is coming out. You may want to have a cold shower after your bath to "clean up!"

TOOL # 8: REST AND FRESH AIR

Rest and fresh air are important when detoxifying. Depending on your life circumstances and daily activities, you may find it helpful to take some time off when you begin to eat instinctively. Applying a twenty-one-day cleanse during your vacation time at the beach or the mountains will give you a tremendous fresh start. If you live in a city, visit a park or the country whenever you can.

TOOL # 9: INSTINCTIVE PHYTOTHERAPY

Herbs, or medicinal plants, can be a valuable aid to detoxination. Ingest strictly unprocessed medicinal plants when there is a pleasant aroma plus salivation. If the aroma is pleasant but there is no salivation, just inhale the aroma. Some examples of when to use herbs are: if detoxination seems sluggish; if there is dissatisfaction after a meal or in the morning; if you are used to eating a big breakfast. You can smell or eat herbs throughout the day, including during meals.

Caution: Herbs available on the market are always dried at high temperature and should not be used for Genefit Nutrition. Dry your own herbs with ventilation only or call The Purefood Network to order a complete set of forty-eight plants or ask for more information.

Even if you have a busy schedule it should be possible to use some of these tools to help your body detoxify and eliminate. In the context of improvement in vitality and well-being, people usually find that they choose what is both enjoyable and effective.

FOURTEEN

Food Supply

Processing Techniques and Treatments

AS ALREADY ADDRESSED in Chapter 6, getting food of the right and truly unprocessed quality is not easy. In order to help you avoid making poor choices, we have made a list with the most common food-processing techniques and treatments currently used. Even if we have tried to make the list as complete as possible, there might be other techniques we have not listed, as treatments are in constant evolution.

1. FRUIT

The major problem with fruit concerns contaminants such as chemical fertilizers, insecticides, abnormal molecules from heated compost and preservatives. Irradiation and waxing are also a problem. Irradiated fruit will not ripen, and its alliesthesial response will be weakened or even nonexistent. If fruit at room temperature for a week or more does not noticeably mature, it may be irradiated. Most fruit in American supermarkets and even health food stores has had its skin sprayed, waxed, or deodorized.

Most imported tropical fruits are subject to chemical and thermal treatments against fruit fly and can therefore not be included in the

Genefit Nutrition food palette. More information about importation regulations is available on the APHIS web site.

Fruits or any other food dried in the sun are not recommended. In most climates, the temperature under full sun exposure at noon exceeds the Genefit quality guidelines and prevents an alliesthesial response in foods so treated.

2. VEGETABLES

Here again a major problem with vegetables is contaminants. Chemical fertilizers, insecticides, and preservative sprays all find their way ultimately into the body of the consumer. Organic fertilizer is sometimes produced with big compost piles where the internal temperature reaches more than 180 degrees. These compost piles will produce abnormal molecules that can then be found in vegetables and fruits. Soaking and washing vegetables is not always recommended since it removes many valuable nutrients and slightly alters taste and smell.

3. DATES

Commercially dried dates are generally dried at high temperature and then frozen. Those dates should be avoided since they can easily be eaten to excess, producing dietary imbalance and discomforts. Dates are often also rehydrated after drying, then washed and eventually glazed with sugar, all of which also prevents a correct alliesthesial response.

4. HONEY

The major problems with honey are extraction by heat, antibiotics, and sugar feeds for bees. "Natural" honey is the only kind there is, so that even when it has been processed industrially, it is still labeled "natural." However, honey is extremely sensitive to heat, and a temperature only a few degrees higher than the one prevailing inside the hive will denature it enough to prevent alliesthesial response.

Honey that is still in the comb is the only truly "natural" honey in a Genefit Nutritional sense. But even then, prior treatment, for instance start-up combs, can prevent a change of taste. It is also natural if it was extracted from the comb by being spooned directly into jars and stored at ambient temperature. A single jar should contain only honey from a single hive. Mixed honey from different hives will not produce a correct alliesthesial response. Industrial honey is inevitably a mixture of honeys, which for the most part were extracted from the comb by melting them. At the factory, the honey will again be heated to liquify it for convenience in mixing, and filling jars or cans. Once treated this way, honey remains relatively fluid; it loses the heavy consistency it would have in its native state. It also loses the ability to produce a proper alliesthesial response: it can be eaten until it makes the eater nauseous, whereas original honey produces a change of taste and/or a burning sensation that prevents excessive ingestion.

Beekeepers who give refined sugar to their bees after removing so much honey that the hive would starve to death otherwise is also a common phenomenon you should be aware of. Some ingenious beekeepers have also been known to feed the bees fruit jams to produce exotic flavors that do not exist in nature. Honey is generally named for some particular type of vegetation, or in a particular environment in which bees feed.

It is always good to have an assortment of honey for testing by smell. It is not a good idea to eat two or three different honeys in quick succession. Even a bottled honey whose label states unequivocally that it is unmixed and unheated above hive temperature should be used with caution, as most treatments are hidden. Bottled honey with a piece of honeycomb floating in it is suspect, particularly if the label gives no explanation.

5. NUTS

The major problems with nuts besides chemical fertilizer and other contaminants are temperature treatments. Nuts available in stores are always frozen and/or heated. Heat is used for fast-drying purposes and frost for conservation. Avoid sun-dried nuts as the temperature is almost always too hot and prevents an accurate alliesthesial response.

Another problem is bleaching. For instance, walnuts from the tree are dark brown, and so in most cases, they have been bleached, giving them a "clean" anemic hue and a deadened, if not patently bitter, taste.

Unless you order nuts from The Purefood Network, you would do well to ask growers about the quality of the nuts they make available.

Shelled "raw" nuts, a favorite in health food stores, are systematically treated and do not produce an accurate alliesthesial response. Here again, you will need to seek out sources of authentic nuts in their original shells, the ones they were "born" in.

6. SEEDS AND LEGUMES

For the most part, these foods are also exposed to the ravages of fertilizers, insecticides, preservatives, shelling processes, and high-temperature drying. Only use seeds and cereals that you can be sure have not been treated. Wheat, soy, and corn are not used in Genefit Nutrition because they synthesize abnormal proteins and do not produce taste changes to signal when the body has enough.

7. MEAT

The most widespread problem with meat comes from what enters the animal's body: chemically fertilized corn or wheat, industrial feeds, cooked slops, synthetic food supplements, synthetic hormones, and vaccines. These additives accumulate in animals' cellular and fatty tissue. The mechanisms of fat accumulation in cattle or pigs reflect those in humans who ingest denatured foods their metabolisms can neither use nor eliminate.

Other common problems come from freezing and selective breeding. When meat ends up cooked anyway it doesn't really matter, but in a Genefit Nutritional referential it prevents an alliesthesial response.

8. EGGS

Commercial eggs from chickens fed commercial fodders, grains, kitchen scraps, etc. should be avoided at any price. Currently there are no eggs on the market matching the quality guidelines required by Genefit Nutrition. Even the so-called organic free-range chickens are fed unnatural foods. Unless you raise your own chickens or order eggs from The Purefood Network, it is not recommend to include them in your food palette.

9. SEAFOOD

The major problems with seafood are freezing and farm raising. Fish in regular retail and health food stores are up to ninety percent frozen, either on the boat or in the wholesaler's processing unit. Commercially grown freshwater and farm-raised saltwater fish, such as salmon, should also be avoided, since they are raised on chemical and processed fodders.

10. POLLEN

The major problems with pollen are extraction by heat and freezing. Pollen is extremely sensitive to temperature changes, and a temperature only a few degrees higher than the one prevailing inside the hive or freezing will denature it enough to prevent a taste change.

After reading all this you are probably asking yourself: "Where do I get my food?" Several options are available to you:

1. Go out on your own. It is not easy, but feasible. Do research, contact growers and farmers, ask food supply companies to find out about the quality of their products.
2. Visit the Purefood web site to get access to a frequently updated list of Purefood certified growers and producers selling Genefit Nutrition-quality foods. Most of them do mail order, so you can order directly online.

3. Order a complete 21-day program package at The Purefood Network, which includes all the food supply necessary for the entire period of the program. One box a week will be sent to the address you provide (see contact information at the end of this book for details).

FIFTEEN

Food Groups
and Meal Sequences

IN THIS CHAPTER, we will discuss the food groups separately along with some of the individual foods within them and how to eat them, as well as make comments about their alliesthesial response.

1. LUNCH

Here is a list of what can be found on a Genefit Nutrition lunch table. These are only a few examples, and your choice doesn't have to be limited to them. Pretty much every food in its truly natural state can be part of your choice. The following remarks do not apply to fruits that have been irradiated or processed in any way:

Group 1: Fruits, Dates, and Honey

Apples   Taste fades or becomes too acidic and texture becomes woody. Overripe apples can be delicious when a person needs them.

Bananas   Both green and overripe bananas may sometimes be more attractive than bananas that seem ideally ripe. At the turning point, taste disappears or becomes grassy.

Berries   Most berries will taste terribly acidic when the body doesn't need them.

Cherries   If you can't smell them, scratch the stem. Taste becomes bland/acid when no longer needed.

Chirimoya   This semitropical fruit is the size of a small muskmelon, with flesh the texture of cream. Superb when the body needs it, becoming somewhat stinky or too sweet when it doesn't. May produce strong detoxination waves in the beginning.

Citrus Fruits   Cut fruit along the equator, then quarter the hemispheres. Let your lips come in contact with the skin, and eat everything inside, including the pith (but not the seeds) to obtain an accurate stop. This applies to all citrus fruits. Always prefer varieties with seeds to seedless ones.

Dates   Many varieties are available. Preferably choose noncommercial varieties instead of the classic barhee, medjool, or deglet noor. Fresh dates become too sweet or too dry (make you thirsty) when no longer needed by the body. It is better to refrigerate dates. They can be stored for a year without problems.

Figs   When no longer needed, fresh figs will burn the mouth. Dried figs from the regular market are always dried at high temperature and should therefore be avoided.

Grapefruit   All varieties can be eaten, but the white-flesh, seed-bearing kind produces the strongest alliesthesial response. See Citrus Fruits.

Grapes   Avoid seedless grapes. In the beginning, scratch the stem to obtain smell. It is recommended to eat the seeds as they are part of the alliesthesial response. Grapes become acid and/or bitter when not needed.

Guava   Sweet when needed, otherwise acid. Can be eaten like an apple, skin and seeds included. With this fruit do not confuse pleasantness of smell and intensity.

Honey   Acacia honey, eucalyptus honey, clover honey, mountain honey, prairie honey, pine forest honey, sagebrush honey, chestnut honey, apple orchard honey, cherry orchard honey, etc. Taste will turn biting, too sweet or burning in the throat at the stop.

Kiwi   This fruit is very sweet when needed, becoming acrid and pungent when enough has been eaten. Kiwis are best eaten cut lengthwise into quarters. Ideally, eat them with the skin or at least let your lips be in contact with the skin.

Kumquats   Can be chewed up and eaten whole, becoming unpleasantly bitter when not needed.

Lemons, Limes   Delicious like grapefruit when needed, becoming acid if not. See Citrus Fruits.

Litchees   Sometimes called the "cherries of Asia." The husk is peeled away, the flesh torn from the single central seed. Highly aromatic, very sweet, changing to sour. Imported litchees are usually treated, per mandatory USDA regulations and so are not recommended.

Mangoes   All mangoes imported into the U.S. are treated with hot steam/hot water as per mandatory USDA regulations. The temperature inside the mango reaches 150 degrees and so these do not match the quality guidelines Genefit Nutrition requires. Avoid!
    Mangoes cultivated by artificial selection have relatively smooth flesh, but have a poor alliesthesial response; root stock mangoes as a rule are smaller and stringy, with more intense smell and taste. Mangoes are best tested by smell where the stalk meets the fruit.

Melons   Watch out for fertilizer aftertaste. Most melons, including watermelons, have a sweet-to-sour or bland taste change. The most hybridized varieties produce a sensation of fullness in the stomach when the stop is reached. Melons are preferably eaten ripe and at room temperature, cut in any way that is convenient.

Nectarines   Because nectarines were first produced by hybridization between peaches and plums, eat them only in ecstatic phase.

Oranges   Many varieties exist, preferences depend on needs. Scratch out spot on skin to obtain stronger smell. See Citrus Fruits.

Papaya   All commercial papayas, even the organic ones, are treated either with chemicals, hot water, or wax due to USDA importation regulations. If you find truly natural papaya, the small varieties can be cut in half lengthwise and eaten with a spoon, with or without the seeds. The smell can get strongly repulsive when the body doesn't need it. Taste changes from delicious to bland.

Passion Fruit   Numerous varieties exist, lemon-sized dark green, orange-sized light yellow, and so on. Fabulously delicious when needed, unbearably acid when the stop-point is reached.

Peaches   All varieties become bland/sour when need has been filled or skin becomes unpleasant. Watch out for excessive artificial selection and hybridization.

Pears   Taste change is usually mild becoming uninteresting or bitter.

Persimmons   Watch out for excessive hybridization; some varieties have a poor alliesthesial response. The well-known puckering effect of persimmons is part of the stop.

Pineapple   The top can be twisted off, and the exposed fruit tested by smell. Pineapples are best cut in half lengthwise, the hemispheres then cut into wedges. Some of the core fiber can be cut off along the top of each wedge, then a series of small perpendicular cuts can be made an inch apart along the wedge to produce convenient bite-size sections to be eaten off the skin. Pineapple produces a ferocious taste change, becoming sharply acid/biting.

Plantain   On a traditional diet this variety of banana is usually used for cooking, but tastes excellent raw to someone who needs it, and is usually eaten when black and soft. Tastes like pancake with jam when the body needs it, but becomes flat-tasting, too sweet, and starchy when need is filled.

Pomegranate   Can be halved or quartered and the seeds picked out in batches with the teeth. Puckers the mouth when the taste change is reached; at this point, beware the temptation to crush and suck seeds for their juice only, which will still taste fairly good.

Plums   All varieties produce a fairly good alliesthesial response, usually an acid increase or loss of flavor. Prunes are dried plums, and are universally heat-dried and produce no taste change and so are to be avoided unless you dry your own. Prunes are not needed to facilitate intestinal passage of foods when a person is eating instinctively.

Natural prunes will not produce diarrhea (i.e., act like "natural laxa-
tives") because they will not be eaten to excess.

Prickly Pears   Watch out for the little spines in the skin, which should
be removed entirely before eating. This fruit is very tasty when
needed, turning bland when the stop-point is reached.

Raisins   Raisins are dried grapes, and are also heat-dried on the market. Same comments as prunes.

Sapote Blanco   Eat with skin when soft. The white flesh is luscious
and incredibly tasty, but becomes biting/bitter when enough has
been eaten.

Tamarind   Small flat shell pulls apart to reveal reddish brown, fudge-
like flesh, with strong pungent odor becoming unbearably acid
when no longer needed. Traditionally used as a laxative, can be
important to unblock constipation when cassia is not sufficient or
creates disgust.

Tomatoes   Highly selected, instinctive stop often blurry. Always prefer
Heirloom varieties.

Watermelon   See Melons.

Commercially grown fruit is artificially bred to taste better to the
"cooked" palate than its wild cousins in nature. Because it takes longer
for the taste to turn bad, we may eat more than we need unless we compensate a little for this factor. The way to do this is to stop eating fruit
when the taste becomes neutral, before it becomes sharply distasteful.
This should be taken as a general rule with fruit in an everyday context.

The argument has been advanced that only locally grown fruits
should be used, and only in season, because this is the natural way of
man's harmony with his environment. This may be relevant for people
who have been on Genefit Nutrition for many years, but for people new
to this way of eating, or people facing serious health conditions, it is very
important to broaden the choice and so give the body maximum
chances to find the food it is precisely looking for. It will save time by
speeding up detoxination and recovery. For some seriously ill people this
can be a matter of life or death.

In general, tropical fruits may be damaged by refrigeration, and should be kept at room temperature, closer to their native ambient temperature. Other fruits can be refrigerated if necessary. Drying fruits in hot air or in the sun will cook them and thus destroy their taste-change potential. Use a simple fan to dry fruit and to keep insects away.

2. DINNER

Dinner starts with a choice of protein-rich and fat-rich foods as a first course, then a choice of vegetables is used for the second course.

The following is a list of what can be found on a Genefit Nutrition dinner table. These are only a few examples and your choice doesn't have to be limited to them. Here again, every food in its truly natural state can be part of your choice. The following remarks do not apply to foods that have been irradiated or processed in any way:

Group 2: High-protein and high-fat foods

Group 2a: Nuts

Almonds   Hard- and soft-shelled varieties.

Brazil nuts   Those available in health food stores are always extracted with heat treatment and should therefore be avoided.

Cashew nuts   Same as Brazil nuts.

Chestnuts   Available in the fall, must be eaten fresh.

Hazelnuts

Peanuts   Fresh peanuts should not be washed.

Pecans

Pistachios   Because of their tendency to mold are always dried at high temperature twenty-four to forty-eight hours after harvest. Make sure the ones you use are not. This holds true also for other varieties of nuts.

Walnuts

Nuts usually turn dry and dusty when the body has no need for them. Take some nuts in the palm of your hand, put them close to your mouth, and blow on them for a few seconds to warm and moisten them and give them an odor. Nuts can be eaten dry when the body needs them or they can be soaked for a few hours first. This makes them more aromatic and sometimes tastier. Nuts, legumes, and seeds are best stored in a dry place at a constant room temperature.

Group 2b: Seafood

Includes clams, mussels, oysters, crabs (all kinds), sardines (all kinds), mackerel, tuna, swordfish, etc.

The taste-change phenomenon varies greatly from one type of seafood to another, and may involve texture as well as taste. Tuna, for example, may become gluey in the mouth and taste like cardboard when the body doesn't need it. Clams, oysters, and other shellfish may become bitter, acrid, or too salty. Scallops may become oversweet, while crab may change from sweet to acrid. The taste change in most seafood occurs rapidly and is clear-cut, probably because animal life from the sea is more truly in its native state, unmodified by selective breeding.

Some people might feel uncomfortable at the idea of eating certain seafood. Remember, with Genefit Nutrition you only eat what smells pleasant and tastes delicious.

Psychological aversions against certain types of food are mostly from cultural origin and can be easily overcome once the taste and smell are extraordinarily pleasant. Japanese sushi bars offer a good example of how broad the food palette can be. Any part of a fish, clam, lobster, or crab can taste delicious when the body needs it.

Larger fish may be rinsed before being cut open, but once they are open it is not recommended to rinse them. The reason is that running water carries away smell, taste, and nutrients. It is better to wipe clean filets or other pieces of fish with a cloth or paper towel if desired.

Do not rinse smaller fish, such as sardines, at all. It will thoroughly alter their smell, and the taste. After the heads and entrails are removed simply wipe the fish clean and lay out on a plate.

Most seafood can be kept fresh for a few days under dry refrigeration (shellfish do not require wrapping). Fish filets can be dried, however, on a coarse mesh at room temperature with a fan. Fish dried this way will still produce an alliesthesial response.

Group 2c: Land animals

Eggs   Eggs can be tested by smell by warming the shell up with your
breath. If the smell of the eggs is attractive, the white and the yolk
can eventually be eaten separately with a spoon. Generally, for the
beginner, the yolk will taste attractive more frequently than the
white. Neither should be eaten unless they are patently delicious.
When the yolk changes taste, it will become bland or sour and the
consistency turn too thick and sticky. The white will taste sweet
when the body needs it, becoming neutral and consistency turning
unpleasant when the need has been filled.

Eggs may be kept in the refrigerator, but it is recommended to eat
them at room temperature.

Meat   Always choose wild game because the selective breeding of
domestic species prevents a clear-cut alliesthesial response. A meat
choice might consist, for instance, of an assortment of venison, antelope, wild boar, pheasant, and hare. When the body needs it, the taste
will mostly be sweet and rich, becoming bitter or flat when one has
had his fill. Unless a piece of meat tastes delicious (not just vaguely
pleasant or acceptable) do not eat it. Ideally, it is best to eat meat by
itself without any additional food. This applies to the meat and organs
of all land animals including fowl. Prepare a few thin slices for
smelling, laid out like cold cuts. Truly natural meat does not spoil as
fast as contaminated meat. When you find the appropriate quality of
meat, you may wish to buy an extra supply to keep on hand. It can be
refrigerated with separate unwrapped pieces hung from wire hooks
(paper clips will work) with space between them for air circulation.
The surface will dry out somewhat, but remain edible.

With time, meat will begin to smell stronger. Persons who regularly eat by instinct will usually find the smell of aged meat more
attractive than the relatively bland odor of fresh meat. Naturally,
what one person might call a stench might be a delight for another.

Here we should remind you that meat is not an absolute necessity,
if you apply the principles of Genefit Nutrition for twenty-one days
only. Not having meat in your palette during that time won't harm
you.

Group 2d: Legumes and Seeds
Beans (all kinds)
Chick Peas
Lentils
Sesame Seeds
Sunflower Seeds
Linseeds (flax)

The taste goes from delicious to grassy or bland. Be aware that even heated or irradiated legumes and seeds are still able to sprout, so this is not a quality guarantee. Any cereal grain except wheat and soy can be used if soaked or sprouted. Legumes can be soaked in water until they are swollen, then eaten like nuts. The seeds most commonly eaten instinctively are sunflower seeds, sesame seeds, and flax seed. They are usually sampled by smell and eaten dry, although they can also be soaked. They are generally attractive in small amounts.

Group 2e: Miscellaneous

Avocado   Many varieties are now available, but watch out for excessive artificial selection and hybridization. In this regard it is recommended to avoid Hass and Fuerte avocados. Always prefer varieties where you can eat the skin. The taste becomes slowly uninteresting and the texture becomes unpleasantly thick as the salivation reflex becomes inactive.

Carob   Natural carob batons can be cut open and chewed if the taste is good. Be aware that this fruit often has a constipating effect, and can be smell-sampled regularly by anyone suffering from loose bowels.

Coconut   Young coconuts available commercially are often bleached to give them a permanent white color, otherwise they quickly turn brown as a result of oxidation just like an apple. It is not recommended to use coconuts so treated. The juice or milk is deliciously sweet when needed and turns bland when stop is reached. In the immature nut, the meat is soft and can be eaten with a spoon, becoming sour when the taste changes. The flesh of a mature coconut can be eaten like that of any other nut, becoming dry when the body has enough.

Smell-sample a coconut by first pulling aside the straw-like hair that often remains over the three "eyes," and then smelling the husk. One of the three eyes is soft, and can easily be pierced with an ice-pick or a knife to insert a straw. Once the milk has been drunk, the coconut can be split by hitting it with a hammer, or by simply throwing it on the floor.

Peas   Sweet and delicious when needed and grassy if not.

Pollen   Taste becomes overwhelmingly strong when stop is reached.

Mushrooms   Do not taste if there is no smell or the smell is unattractive. Do not peel mushrooms. Taste changes to neutral or variably distasteful depending on variety. Stop eating as soon as this occurs. Absolutely avoid poisonous varieties if untrained nutritional instinct.

Olives   Eat when black and wrinkly. Taste turns terribly bitter when they are no longer needed. Olives offered on the market are usually conserved in oil and spices. Only cold-dried, unseasoned, uncured olives can be used.

Group 3: Vegetables

Artichokes   Only the base of the leaves and the heart are usually eaten. Cut lengthwise into quarters. Remove the fuzz from the heart. Eat the bases of the leaves, working toward the heart. They are fabulously delicious when the body needs them, but former consumers of cooked artichokes may not find raw ones attractive for some time. Sharp, rapid taste change from delicious to piquant or bitter.

Asparagus   The stem and the flower can be eaten. Taste slowly becomes sour.

Broccoli   Sometimes people need the florets, and sometimes the stalks are the right food. Broccoli becomes burning when stop occurs.

Brussels Sprouts   Sweet and sour taste when needed, becoming very sour or burning.

Cabbage   Both red and green cabbages are fine. The base of the leaf is tastiest. Deliciously sweet when needed, becoming hot when not.

Cauliflower   Same comments as broccoli.

Celeriac (celery root)   Becomes very sharp when no longer needed.

Celery   Strong taste change. Becomes intolerable at taste change.

Chinese Cabbage   When not needed becomes bitter or "tastes like cardboard."

Corn   Caution: artificial selection and genetic engineering. Avoid.

Cucumbers   Do not peel. Becomes acrid when no longer needed. Watch out for waxing even from health food stores.

Eggplant   Most people never find raw eggplant attractive, but some swear by it. Tastes like "plaster" when not needed.

Garlic   If the smell is strongly attractive, enjoy the smell until it subsides or turns bad. It is providing valuable aromatic nutrition. Suck on it carefully when salivation reflex occurs and the taste is mild. Spit it out immediately when the taste becomes hot, which means the body doesn't need it any longer.

Jicama   Changes from a mild sweet taste to a pungent earthy flavor at the stop.

Kohlrabi   Pleasant taste becomes unpleasantly strong with a fairly fast transition.

Leeks   The same comments as garlic: smell only if no salivation. Green and white parts can be eaten. Leek taste change is phenomenally rapid so spit it out as soon as it occurs.

Lettuce   From a juicy or even oily taste sensation to uninteresting, slightly sour or bitter taste at change.

Mint   Crush leaves in your fingers and enjoy the smell for a while before tasting. Becomes bitter when not needed.

Okra   Same comments as eggplant.

Parsley   Crush in your fingers to test by smell. If salivation reflex occurs, taste. Parsley becomes biting when no longer needed.

Parsnips   Fairly fast taste change to unbearably strong.

Peppers   Red, green, and yellow bell peppers are aromatic and very different from one another. They become bitter when not needed. Hot peppers become too hot when the taste changes.

Potatoes Most conveniently eaten in slices. If you aren't overloaded from a long history of cooked potatoes you will find them very attractive on occasion. Sweet and creamy when needed by the body reverting to a "raw potato" taste when not needed.

Pumpkin Sweet, almost like melon, when needed, but pumpkins become sticky when stop occurs.

Radishes If the taste is mildly but pleasantly biting, keep going, but stop when bite becomes strong.

Rhubarb Aromatic sweetness becoming piquant.

Rutabaga Becomes sour/biting when not needed.

Spinach Will become sour and puckering when not needed.

Squash Same comments as eggplant.

Turnips Become sour and biting when not needed.

Watercress Same comments as parsley.

Yams Best eaten like potatoes. Delicious for people who need them, otherwise they are unpleasantly bland or dry.

Zucchini Same comments as eggplant.

It is preferable to eat vegetables at room temperature. It is recommended to smell-sample them by scratching or making a cut in the skin first.

Problems may arise as a result of artificial selection. In their efforts to increase profits, growers have for many years been developing special strains of produce designed to stand up better during shipment, resist parasites, and be visually more attractive. They have also sought to enhance a bland flavor in varieties that are normally eaten raw like cucumbers and tomatoes. These are the ones that sell best, because weak vegetables produce weak alliesthesial responses, and consumers therefore eat more of them.

Vegetables destined for cooking, on the other hand, are artificially selected for their attractiveness after cooking. The result is that most raw vegetables on the market are less attractive than they would be if they had never been tampered with. They are relatively so unattractive, in fact, that unless we know how to compensate for it, we may end up eating so few that we deprive ourselves of nutrients that only vegetables can provide. Fancy dressings are not the answer. If we can, we need to account for the calculated imbalance of vegetables, and it is easy to do so once we understand how our taste change works in relation to them.

It was mentioned earlier that fruits are raised to be more attractive than they would be in nature, so it is best to stop when their taste becomes mildly good, before it goes flat or bad. But, as a result of artificially selection, vegetables are unnaturally less attractive when raw, so the opposite applies. In other words, eat vegetables not until the neutral point is reached, but until the taste has become clearly unpleasant.

Vegetables keep best if refrigerated, but wrapping them in plastic is not the best way to store them. Unless they can breathe they will begin to rot, and they will wither unless they are kept moist. Some health food stores carry plastic bags with perforations specially designed for vegetable storage.

SIXTEEN

What to Expect

GENEFIT NUTRITION is the most thorough and comfortable way to detoxify or cleanse your body. When the body is given the opportunity to choose food instinctively, it is able to take all possible factors into account, including repair, maintenance, strengthening, and the elimination of stored waste. Your body will have its particular priorities, and it will naturally commence its optimizing program at a pace that all systems can handle. Some cleansing programs bypass the body's own capabilities by stimulating a "dumping" of toxins into the system, which can cause severe physical, mental, and emotional trauma.

When eating instinctively however, the body is able to choose food specific to its needs, so the processes of detoxination experienced are often "silent." That is, the body is cleaning up and getting things in order, but there may be little or no discomfort. However, it is always a good idea to know all of the possible scenarios, so let's take a look at the Three Steps of Detoxination and see what could happen.

STEP ONE: EXCHANGE

Natural molecules from unprocessed food chosen instinctively, taken in by the body, wake up the immune system, which then encourages cells to give up their stored toxins. Cells will continue to store harmful substances until they are either forced to dislodge them or, preferably, it is safe to dislodge them as something better comes along. From the time you eat your first instinctive meal you cause a phenomenon of exchange to occur in the cells of your body; that is, the cells exchange stored waste for quality nutrients.

Unfortunately, if your former diet normally consisted of processed foods, the cells will have a level of waste that is unnatural. From this polluted medium the cell must do the best it can to fulfill its functions. Conventional "slimming" diets do not produce lasting, sustainable results because the body is either not getting anything to stimulate exchange or it is just getting a different version of processed foods. Unfortunately, there is usually dissatisfaction and frustration with conventional diets, followed by a return to the "old ways" of eating.

STEP TWO: POTENTIAL DISCOMFORT

Toxins have moved out of the cells but are still in the body. As the toxins are dislodged from their storage in the cells, they will be picked up by the lymph capillaries and vessels and eliminated by several means (bowel, kidneys, skin, and lungs). If you are using your Toolbox there may be little or no discomfort at this stage. However, if your means of elimination are sluggish, the toxins will tend to sit around in the bloodstream, joints, interstitial spaces, and bowel.

There are many possible manifestations at this stage due to the variety of toxins that can be present. When eating instinctively these manifestations of detoxination can turn into slight symptoms, which usually pass quickly as the toxins are eliminated from the body. They are not truly pathologic because the detoxination process is part of an improvement in well-being. Detoxination is followed by an improvement in physical condition, signifying repair and increased efficiency on a cellular level. You will look and feel noticeably better. When Genefit Nutrition is applied correctly detox waves typically pass quickly and are mild in nature.

Cravings, dreams, restlessness, and vivid memories of processed food smells and tastes can all manifest when the body is in a detoxination cycle. This is the time when you will be most tempted to give in, quit, "just have one little piece," or yell at someone! There really isn't a magic pill, or "quick fix," except to understand what is happening when you are in it, and do the best you can to get the body through that particular detoxination cycle (see Chapter 13).

STEP THREE: ELIMINATION

Toxins are leaving the body; say goodbye to the cause of problems! The manifestations of detoxifying may be uncomfortable at times. The discomfort is present because the body is getting rid of what it considers harmful or useless and will cease when the process is complete. The fact that the body is able to detoxify indicates progress and improvement towards a new level of health. A "silent" detoxination, characterized by minimal discomfort, is common when one follows the guidelines of the instinct. Repeated symptoms may be an indication of an error. Check to see if you are using the principles fully, leaving something out or adding something in. If troubles persist we strongly recommend contacting us.

Genefit Nutrition is a technology that has been developed over decades of research, practice, and observation. The mechanism of instinct can be either listened to or bypassed. It gives hundred percent results when used a hundred percent of the time. Adding other practices for faster, better results interferes with the body's programs and inhibits understanding of symptoms.

The detoxination of altered and unaltered molecules can be observed to occur at different times during the day and night. The body normally detoxifies the natural waste of the metabolism shortly after midnight. Generally speaking this cycle, which is totally symptom free, lasts through the night, and on its completion one should wake refreshed and feeling cleansed. However, if the body is toxic with abnormal molecules, another cycle will follow. This second cycle lasts from about six a.m. until the first meal or, if the body is heavily loaded with toxins, may last throughout the day.

There are no shortcuts to detoxifying, however using tools such as cassia, movement, and water will be a big help to your body. These are your means of elimination; if you don't use them things will slow down, clog up, and cause discomfort. It is often not helpful to the body to apply any of the many therapies designed to suppress symptoms. We are not callously suggesting that people should have to put up with pain; rather, to recognize what's going on and use the Toolbox to help your body eliminate what is becoming dislodged and to ensure your detoxination goes smoothly through its cycle, with no pain.

DETOXIFYING AND WEIGHT

The results of detoxifying by eating instinctively are spectacular. You can expect a more toned, vibrant, vital body and experience greater confidence, energy, well being, mental clarity, intuition, creativity, and enjoyment of life.

You will lose excess fat and build and tone muscle. Your weight loss will depend on the degree of toxicity, the body's pace of detoxination, and how well you apply the formula.

An application of ninety-five percent does not equal ninety-five percent results. On average you may experience a steady weight loss of half a pound to a pound a day, which may suddenly stop and then resume a few days later.

Fat is a storehouse for toxins. The body may be slowing down the detoxination of some of the more harmful stored substances. Weight loss can be the greatest area of concern and interference from the intellect. For example, if there is anxiety over weight loss one can push past an instinctive stop and eat more. Unfortunately, the cells then exchange out more toxins causing more weight loss. This vicious cycle is easily avoided by accurately following the principles of eating instinctively. If you don't eat enough in a meal there will be more attraction in the next meal. It is a trap of the old paradigm that more food equals more strength. The strength of the body will depend on its ability to use nutrients, the integrity and competency of its systems, and the mental and spiritual state of the individual.

Each of us will have our own idea of how much weight we might want to lose or gain and how quickly we would like to reach our optimum body shape. As the body detoxifies it may go through several shape and appearance changes. When you begin to eat instinctively these changes are associated with detoxifying. After a while your body will start to show the effects of receiving the nutrients it needs by the means of increased muscle tone, clear eyes, good skin, and a sense of vitality. It is important to be confident in your instinct, knowing that by eating instinctively your body will find and maintain its ideal weight.

The limited intellect doesn't have the mechanisms to balance health, but the infinitely sophisticated mechanism of instinct does. Intellect should enhance instinct and vice versa, because together they can be quite a team.

YOU AND YOUR PSYCHOLOGY

Genefit Nutrition is different from the current existing food paradigm. Our cultural habits, ideas, beliefs, comforts, and securities are deeply interwoven with our culinary culture. Food means much more than just nutrition. It is linked with love, sex, agreement, admiration, obedience, control, belonging, reward, indulgence, and self-destruction. Our very identity of who we are contains food likes, dislikes, events, recipes, and restaurants. To suddenly be outside that paradigm can be an unsettling experience. Practicing and planning Genefit Nutrition in limited time segments of for instance three or twenty-one days is the best way to deal with these psychological challenges.

AFTER 21 DAYS

As per fasting, if you have decided to go with Genefit Nutrition for longer than a week, a slow transition is needed once you have decided to revert back to a traditional diet. Now that you have detoxified your body, increased your sensitivity to toxic molecules, and awakened your immune system, your way back to the culinary arts (or artifice) should definitely be gradual.

The best way to proceed is to follow the steps of our human evolutionary history of food processing—although, of course, you will do it a little faster. If you proceed this way it will allow you to introduce the less toxic foods first and the more toxic ones last. The simplest form of processing is mixing, so start with salads. Go to the next step only if your body feels comfortable with the current one. The next step may be steamed vegetables. Stick with steamed vegetables for the time needed to stabilize your body system again. A following step is carbohydrate-rich foods such as cooked potatoes, beans, sweet potatoes, and rice. Next are cooked animal proteins. Finally, introduce dairies, wheat, corn, soy, and their by-products last. If you take these gradual steps you will slowly allow your body to tolerate processed food again. Nothing hinders you from doing another 21-day cleanse later. Even if you aren't able to enjoy the full benefits of Genefit Nutrition all the time, you can still profit from its preventive virtues several times a year. For those who cannot apply Genefit Nutrition all the time, off program we recommend the way of eating defined by Harvey and Marilyn Diamond in their bestseller *Fit for Life*.

THE SOCIAL ASPECTS

In most societies and cultures, the odds are in favor of the cooked food scenario. There are not many Genefit restaurants — yet. So, you may come up against some interesting social challenges when you are eating instinctively, e.g., what to order at an important business lunch.

Many conventional restaurants sometimes agree to make a choice of fruits or unprocessed vegetables available. Also, eating your instinctive meal before you go can save you from being hungry when you are out so your choices will then be more determined.

Genefit Nutrition is certainly a change in eating which can also affect other aspects of life. You may find yourself taking a fresh look at long agreed-upon social "rituals" and subsequently taking great delight in "throwing out the old and bringing in the new."

We do urge compassion for your friends however, who may only see that they have lost you to a strange new food cult!

It helps if your partner is also eating instinctively, or at least is supportive and respectful of your choices, as you should be of theirs. Genefit

Nutrition is both physiologically and psychologically a new paradigm. By applying the principles, and being prepared for what can manifest, it is a means of addressing many issues, which will give greater freedom and capacity for enjoyment of life. The determining factors will be your goals, circumstances, and priorities.

Whatever your decisions, enjoy yourself — and good luck!

PART FOUR

Food, Health, and Illness

In general, people who have seen in serious health issues a spiritual wake-up call to change their lives have been more likely to achieve recovery. As you will see in the following testimonials, for people who choose Genefit Nutrition, reconsidering not only dietary habits, but also many other fields of their life increased their chances of success. Since Genefit Nutrition affects people on more profound levels, it cannot be applied as a regular treatment in itself — a more radical change of life is necessary to fully profit from its benefits.

SEVENTEEN

Food and Allergies

IN ORDER TO UNDERSTAND how Genefit Nutrition works, let us begin by looking at the bewildering problem of allergy, usually termed a "disorder." This description implies that, if you suffer from it, something is wrong with you. Obviously something is wrong, but as you will see, not with you. The current medical model for allergies assumes that the body has, for unknown reasons, become hypersensitive to some foreign substance (an allergen) to which it overreacts, and that further inputs of the allergen will further increase the organism's sensitivity and reactions, and so on, indefinitely. It follows, logically, that attempts should therefore be made to:

1. avoid the allergen,
2. decrease the sensitivity to it and/or
3. suppress reactions to it.

In point of fact, your body is sensitive to *any* incoming substance whose antigenic marking is foreign. This is what triggers (or should trigger) the production of antibodies that will destroy the "alien" and eliminate it from your body. Therefore, to whatever degree 2) and/or 3) above are successful, they are, to that degree, dangerous for your long-term integrity. Suppressing the reactions artificially may produce apparent (usually temporary) relief, but will eventually hinder the immune system from doing its work.

Allergens are detonators, but they are not the gunpowder. Allergic reactions are protective reactions. They are natural. Normally, they occur wherever alien material touches the body's "surface." Normally, they should be confined to the sole site of the allergen's point of contact (e.g., the nasal epithelium, the intestinal wall, etc.). And normally, the reactions should end there, their number limited to the number of allergens. And that is the way it would happen, but for the prior accumulation in the body of nutritional toxins whose structure is similar to the allergen.

Nutritional toxins have previously accumulated because the immune system did not recognize them as foreign, did not respond with attempts to eliminate them, or did not succeed in doing so.

When this has occurred the immune system is said to be in a state of tolerance.

An immunologic state of tolerance is, in many regards, an unstable state. It can be disrupted either by unnatural allergens (nylon, latex, shampoo, etc.) or mostly by natural allergens, such as pollen, fruits, peanuts, or seafood. Because of the presence of such huge amounts of accumulated abnormal molecules in the body, the immune system is always bouncing from tolerance to intolerance and vice versa, depending on many internal and external factors — allergens are external factors.

When the chemical structure of the allergen is similar to that of a specific class of abnormal molecules that has accumulated in the body, contact with that allergen can, if several conditions are reunited, break the state of tolerance. It will then recognize and eliminate the allergen together with chemically similar abnormal molecules. In other words, a person can only be "allergic" to molecular structures similar to the nutritional toxins he is already loaded with.

For example, let's say you're a bread-eater, a consumer of heat-processed chemical compounds of wheat, which were alien to humankind's native alimentary spectrum even before being baked. After repeated exposure to bread in early childhood, your body became perfectly tolerant of it. As a result, your cells have become loaded with the wheat's abnormal proteins. Now, it is summer, and a microscopic bit of chaff or pollen from wheat or some other grass comes into contact with a cell in your nasal epithelium. Normally, a secretion should occur at that site, to isolate and rinse away the pollen, and it still does. But instead of limiting its response to a few actual bits of invasive pollen, the body responds as well to the vast, accumulated deposits of the grasses-type impurities that came from your daily bread. They are still there, stuck in your cells. So instead of a minor, imperceptible secretion from a few cells alone, a chain reaction starts, and millions of cells begin to isolate and rinse away the foreign wheat-like material they had been putting up with. Out comes your handkerchief.

As long as you continue to eat bread or wheat products, you will be prey to hay fever. The accumulation levels in your cells will vary, and so will your degree of tolerance, but when conditions are right, you will experience hay fever. If you keep on eating bread or wheat products, you will have accumulated enough to set the stage for another massive "allergic" detoxination crisis.

If the symptoms of "allergy" vary greatly, it is probably because our diets include such a wide variety of unidentified poisons. An "allergic" reaction reflects an attempt to eliminate them. But toxins being ejected from the cells must pass through the bloodstream on their way out. In doing so, they can produce cramps, diarrhea, headaches, drowsiness, coughing, sneezing, uticaria, dizziness, palpitations, sweating, watering eyes, and altered emotional states, including unwarranted fears, anger, and depression.

The reason these symptoms are called "allergies" in the first place is that they occur in response to substances that would normally be considered innocuous, in contrast to recognized toxins. No one is said to be "allergic" to toadstools or bad oysters but if someone reacts strongly to strawberries (which are not supposed to be toxic), then he is said to be "allergic" to them. Persons who react strongly to bread, fried potatoes, and other foods are described as *abnormal* (i.e., they have a food allergy), because those foods are considered *normal* foods for humans. In fact, they are *not* at all normal for our species, as we have learned.

All this happens because of the mis-metabolized accretions from denatured food that disrupts our organic harmony, which is in itself the most basic cause of disease. Once your body has been cleaned out, so that it is no longer permeated with debris, there is nothing it needs to get rid of. It won't need to undertake a general housecleaning when invaded by a few irritants at specific sites. Dust and smoke will still provoke coughing, watery eyes, a washing away of the irritant, as they should. But there the reactions will stop, because there is no need for them to occur, except locally.

Not only does Genefit Nutrition provide automatic relief from symptoms of allergies of all kinds, it turns allergies into something useful. Under Genefit Nutrition eating conditions, every time a detoxination wave takes place, it is thanks to an allergic (or similar) reaction triggered by the consumption of an unprocessed food, which simply breaks the state of tolerance. If you eat the kinds and amounts of the foods you truly need, and for which you were biochemically constructed, you will spontaneously rid yourself of the toxins gathered from your denatured nutritional past. For a time, your body will periodically smell strongly, as it discharges unusable residues from the stews, soups, snacks, and seasonings you consumed over the years, until you become close to odorless. At that point, allergic reactions will have become impossible — along with inflammatory pain, fungus, bacterial infections, and many other conditions.

Can these claims be proven? You will see for yourself, once you have learned to trust your instinct. They will become self-evident, at the cost of giving up a few traditions, habits, and taboos. All you have to do is obey the innate wisdom and felt demands of your own body, in preference to catalogued prescriptions designed to treat symptoms instead of their cause.

NAME: Lisa S.

YEAR OF BIRTH: 1970

As a child and throughout my adolescence, I had been dealing with severe acne and sun allergies which got worse every year. My body's ability to heal was very slow with a high tendency to inflammation and scar formation. What had been sunburns as a child transformed into a full-blown allergy by the age of seventeen. Ten to thirty minutes in the sun, depending on its intensity, was enough to cause terrible itching even before my skin turned red. These crises sometimes lasted for several days. Sun creams only irritated my skin and I resigned myself to always wearing long-sleeve shirts and long pants even on the hottest summer days, both to protect myself from the sun and to hide my acne and scars. The summer before I discovered Genefit Nutrition, I was sitting on the beach on the Spanish Atlantic coast covered completely with clothing from head to toe. Although my skin is quite fair, it did not seem normal to me to be so extremely sensitive to the sun, even if people were telling me that it might be related to the increasing holes in the ozone layer.

After my vacation in Spain, I began eating instinctively and rapidly observed ameliorations on my skin. Although it took months until my face and back were totally clear of acne, the inflammatory tendency disappeared, allowing rapid healing. The following summer, encouraged by other testimonials, I dared a little sun exposure. Amazingly, there was no itching anymore. Only when I pushed it to the limit did I end up with a little sunburn. My skin peeled but even that wasn't painful at all. By the end of the summer, I realized that most of my scars had disappeared as if they had been pealed away with the sunburn. I learned to listen to my body to find the right amount of sun exposure, almost like listening to an instinctive stop during a meal.

A few years later, I spent several weeks in Southeast Asia on the beach and in the mountains without any bad experiences, and even without using any sunblock or cream. I simply listened to the signals of my body.

Acne, other than during some psychologically challenging moments, has not been a problem anymore. My thirst for sun has increased over the years and rather than being afraid of it, I appreciate its nurturing and healing effects. Genefit has given me a feeling of freedom and self-confidence I had never known before.

Lisa S.

EIGHTEEN

Food and Cancer

CANCER CELLS are mutant cells produced — to a small extent — naturally by the body. They are normally destroyed by the immune system as soon as they appear. Carcinogenic and mutagenic molecules contained in processed food boost the production of cancer cells to an abnormal level. In addition, as already noted in Chapter 10, when processed food is regularly consumed, the immune system is already in a generalized state of tolerance; it has become passive to abnormal proteins. If abnormal molecules tolerated by the immune system are of similar nature to the ones constituting cancer cells, not only are abnormal molecules no longer destroyed and eliminated, but neither are cancer cells allowing them to proliferate and create tumors. There is no devilish agent that makes cells cancerous; they become that way themselves. The relationship between abnormal food and cancer is strongly supported by an increasing number of highly reputable studies:

> Epidemiological studies have shown a relationship between several types of human cancer, such as esophageal, breast, and colon, and particular kinds of diet, indicating the presence of carcinogenic factors in those diets. Observations in animals have shown that some types of cancer in them are related to certain carcinogens in their food. Several types of cancer similar to that in humans have been induced in experimental animals by administration of carcinogens, such as nitrosamines and mycotoxins, suggesting that their presence in human diets can increase cancer risk. The search for such car-

cinogens, and for others presently unsuspected in human diets, should be continued with the objective of reducing or eliminating human exposure to them. The role of promoting agents, such as fats, in colon and breast cancer needs to be further investigated, and exposure to them should be reduced. Two sources of carcinogens that need increased study are the formation of carcinogens in cooking, especially of fats and proteins, and the endogenous formation of carcinogens in the gastrointestinal tract, e.g., N-nitroso compounds (W. Lijinsky, *Summation and new approaches to diet and cancer.* Cancer Res 1983 May;43[5 Suppl]:2441s-2443s).

From the Genefit Nutritional viewpoint, it is clearly agreed that denatured or even undigested nutrients play a major role in the etiology of all types of cancers.

"The right kind of diet might help reduce the number of dietary cancers. Such nutritional advice is backed up by epidemiological surveys and, as yet, limited though promising experiments on animals." Within the evolutionary time span, human diet has very recently altered and very fast at that. Anthropological investigations of human diet in twentieth-century hunter-fruit pickers like the Kalahari Desert Bushmen in South Africa distill a clear picture of evolution in human diet and the possible impact of dietary changes. On the basis of collated data, Boyd Eaton and Malvin Konner of Emory University infer that prehistoric men living under temperate climes ate 20 percent of their intake in fats. This amounts to approximately half the amount Americans eat. Moreover, prehistoric men ate proportionately more unsaturated fats than we do. They ate around 45 grams of fiber a day (as compared to Americans, who eat 15 grams or less) and four times as much vitamin C. If modern man (*Homo sapiens*) well and truly appeared on Earth some 30-50,000 years ago, for upwards of 90 percent of his history, the human race has eaten a vitamin C, calcium-, fiber-rich diet, which was also a low-fat one. In other words, modern man is now eating out of step metabolically and digestively as compared to the way he used to eat. The fruit-picking hunters' diet still endured (incorporating only minor changes when agriculture came on the scene about 10,000 years ago) up until 250 years ago. At the time, the Industrial Revolution worked a thorough change into human dietary patterns. People started eating more fat, less roughage, more refined sugar and fewer starchy carbohydrates. We are saying that modern man's diet is abnormal. His prehistoric physiology has to make do with a grossly unsuitable diet. It is suspected that dietary changes connected to a sedentary lifestyle have given a boost to the size of the human frame, but have also nudged up obesity, fast maturation in young people and chronic diseases like coronary thrombosis and cancer. Those diseases occurred less commonly even in the elderly in Western culture in the eighteenth and nineteenth centuries and are still almost unheard of in present-day fruit-picking hunters. (L. Cohen, *Diet and cancer.* "In Favor of Science," Jan. 1988, p. 20.)

After Genefit Nutrition progressively reactivates the body's immune sensitivities, the immune system will be able to:

1. generate detoxination processes eliminating accumulated carcinogenic and mutagenic molecules, and
2. recognize and destroy cancerous cells, and so eliminate the tumors.

If food can cause cancer, doesn't it seem reasonable to expect that food might also cure it?

Biochemical experiments performed at the Imperial College of Medicine and the Institute of Food Research support the largely epidemiological link between a diet rich in cruciferous vegetables and lowered risk of developing colon cancer.[2] Cooking meat induces the formation of heterocyclic aromatic amines (HAs), which, when metabolized in the liver, release carcinogens. Vegetables produce glucosinolates, which activate enzymes that detoxify HAs ("In Cancer Research, Diet and Exercise Roles Strengthen," *The Scientist* 15[20]:17, Oct. 15, 2001).

NAME: Maria L.

YEAR OF BIRTH: 1948

Luckily, nature does not always follow the prognosis of physicians. Otherwise, I would no longer be alive.

In the fall of 1994, I became more and more aware that my general health was deteriorating. I was always tired, easily caught colds, I suffered from allergies, inflammation of the small intestine, and severe pain in my left foot.

October 31, 1994, I was diagnosed with a cancerous tumor the size of a beer glass, four inches between the large intestine and the uterus, in the Douglas space. I was hospitalized in the Universitaetsklink Benjamin Franklin in Berlin on November 1, 1994. Six doctors examined my situation and the computer-assisted tomography confirmed to within eighty percent the suspicion that I was dealing with a fast-growing malignant cancer. A definitive diagnosis could only be given with a histological examination.

To save my life, surgery was highly recommended. As the cancer was close to several important organs there was a risk that some would have to be taken out. The eventual necessity of an artificial large intestine exit was also mentioned. No alternative healing approaches were discussed, even after exhaustive discussions with my doctor who told me that those who tried alternative healing approaches were no longer alive.

Realizing what life after the surgery would be like, I decided against it. On November 3, I finally left the hospital exhausted.

The University clinic had a good reputation and the doctors seemed to be qualified. I was happy that they had been so honest with me. However I still had the impression that surgery was not the solution for me.

On November 5, I started eating instinctively with a friend.

During the first weeks, my health condition seemed to become rather worse than better: I lost even more weight and became extremely weak. But slowly I began to regain some strength and after four months, on February 28, 1995, the ultrasound testing of the same hospital in Berlin confirmed that the tumor had disappeared. The doctors could not find any valid explanation.

After seven years of instinctive eating with exclusively unprocessed foods, I feel great and actually weigh twelve pounds more than before the cancer.

I owe my life to this way of eating and the group of people teaching it. I recommend it to everyone, and wish that not only people suffering from severe diseases will discover the fun, the satisfaction, and the positive changes that one can experience thanks to Genefit Nutrition.

Maria L.

NAME: Kamilla H.
YEAR OF BIRTH: 1955

It was Easter 1999 that I discovered that a so-far harmless cyst had become much bigger. During the mammogram and medical examination that followed, my physician showed me the image of the inch-square knot in my breast. He recommended a biopsy (tissue analysis) and warned me up front that if the tumor was malignant, it would have to be surgically removed right away. The situation required immediate action because a punctured breast cancer would diffuse easily with the tendency to create metastasis that could possibly reach the ribs and heart.

The diagnosis was a big shock: malignant breast cancer. The doctor urged me to have the surgery five days later. The idea of having surgery made me panic and at first I was unable to think clearly. Pictures of scars, bald heads, and weeks of nausea and eventually a premature death occupied my mind.

Then a friend involved in alternative healing approaches reassured me that I would survive even if I did not have the surgery immediately, and that there was enough time to look for other options. An intense period of research followed as I tried to find people who had been healed from cancer using alternative approaches.

As all doctors agreed on urgently recommending surgery, my fear persisted.

The turning point came when one of my doctors said that while preparing for surgery it wouldn't really matter how I was feeling the day of surgery because I would be anesthetized anyway and so vulnerably exposed on the operating table. Later, I wondered if this was the often-described cynical physician who finally wanted to get rid of me. Maybe my protective angel had put those words into his mouth, but anyway it was the straw that broke the camel's back. As a little ritual, I burned the transfer papers for the surgery and decided to only listen to my heart from now on.

Many friends had advised me not to do the surgery, and by that time I had found out about a woman who had been cured of a similar cancer with a method of eating by instinct within a few months, and without any other medication. I immediately decided to try the method.

At first, I lost about ten pounds, weighing only 42kg (92 lbs.). But after four months, I found out that the cancer had disappeared.

One year later, I keep getting more and more healthy by continuing eating instinctively. I actually feel more fit than ever before. The wrinkles on my face have disappeared and my friends tell me that I look five years younger. For the first time in my life I have been able to gain some weight and with a height of 168cm (5'6"), I now weigh 52kg (114 lbs.). The knot in my breast hasn't reappeared.

Back in Berlin, I moved to a little house close to the edge of the town to be able to live a more natural life. There have been many other changes in my life and this exciting process is continuing. I know now that miracles are possible when you believe in and respect the harmony of nature.

I also know that it is possible to get rid of cancer while experiencing profound eating pleasure if you are ready to learn from what is happening inside you and to take your life in your own hands. But, you need to be ready to change it drastically and to follow your instinct and nature.

Kamilla H.

NINETEEN

Food and Autoimmune Disease

IN THE CASE OF CANCER, the immune system has "fallen down on the job," and has failed to prevent the spread of abnormal, alien cells. In autoimmune disease, just the opposite has happened: the immune system has gone crazy and is attacking the body's own cells. How can this happen? Normally, the immune system would attempt to destroy and eliminate only matter alien to it. It seems, therefore, if normal cells are attacked, it must be because they have been identified as alien. And how could such mistaken identity occur?

Once we have understood that abnormal molecules from denatured or unnatural foods do, in fact, accumulate in the body, we can see how, in some cases, the cells themselves (and not only the residues they contain) might become targets for destruction. If certain conditions are met, abnormal molecules deposit on the cell's membrane. Every cell in the body carries some kind of I.D.: its membrane displays specific proteins for the immune system to recognize. If the proteins on the membrane mark the cell as being part of the body, it is not attacked. But if the proteins on the membrane are alien, the immune system attacks and destroys the cell. When abnormal, undigested proteins deposit on the cell's membrane, they can overwrite the cell's marker proteins, and the cell itself is then viewed as being foreign, even if it is a perfectly healthy body cell. Such a cell is dealt with as someone would be if his identity tag were overwritten with the name of a dangerous terrorist. In this case, it is likely he would not pass any airport's security control. If things get tense, the police might shoot him, even if, in reality, he is a perfectly peaceful citizen. This is the picture shown by autoimmune diseases.

When persons with autoimmune diseases begin practicing Genefit Nutrition, their immune systems reawaken and become increasingly intolerant of toxic residues in the body, and odors appear from unnatural foods eaten in the past. In autoimmune cases, the odors almost invariably suggest putrid dairy products. This is often true in cancer cases as well. Next, the person's condition may worsen temporarily, as his immune system becomes more vigorous and intolerant of alien introjects (for it has been identifying whole cells as alien, not just part of their content). Great care must be exercised in treating autoimmune disease to ensure detoxination proceeds at a slow, steady pace. Fortunately, you can regulate your own detoxination quite simply by precisely following the signals of your nutritional instinct. After some weeks or months, the danger of uncontrolled self-destruction passes. Once the targeted cells have become sufficiently cleansed of abnormal molecules, the immune system ceases identifying them as "alien." When this happens, and immune responses become focused on nutritional toxins contained in cells, but not on entire cells, regeneration can begin.

Improvement may be irregular, occurring in waves. But as long as Genefit Nutrition is strictly adhered to, no setback should be worse than the one before it. This assumes, of course, that when the practice of Genefit Nutrition was started, irreversible damage had not yet occurred; that is, the pathology had not reached a point of no return. But even where the degenerative process can only be arrested, people are spared further deterioration. Significantly, a number of people suffering from autoimmune disease on the road to recovery have reported that worse-than-last-time relapses would occur if they strayed from careful instinctive practice — but only if and when they did so.

NAME: Dominique G., sailor and writer

YEAR OF BIRTH: 1956

Until 1985, I was sailing and practicing apnea diving intensively. At the beginning of 1985, I first experienced symptoms of tiredness with loss of muscular weight, elocution problems, and diverse paralysis in the legs and arms. In May 1985, I experienced a second crisis with facial hemiplegia (partial paralysis), diplopia (double vision), and severe fatigue. Multiple sclerosis was diagnosed. Then in 1986, I had yet additional strong crises with total loss of sight in my left eye for three weeks. Partial (thirty percent) recovery of sight returned in three months.

I started eating instinctively in 1987.

The first day, I literally devoured four pounds of meat! At dinner that night, I had still more meat. The second day was pretty much the same as the first one. The third day at sunset, I realized that I hadn't experienced any headaches during the entire day. I even forgot to take my medication. I had been living on pain medication for years. It was amazing, only a few days after the beginning of my practice, I observed a total disappearance of the strong headaches that had made my life so difficult during the past two years.

On the morning of the fifth day, my eye perceived a new universe. I couldn't believe it. Every three minutes I closed the other eye to test if I was right. My sight was improving rapidly. During the day, I did not notice an improvement, but every morning when I woke up, I saw the improvement.

On the eighth day, I cleaned the kitchen of my boat, the *Poisson Lune*. I put all my little kitchen accessories out on the deck and decided to get rid of them. Over the weeks, many of these cooking accessories left the boat to join the ocean or make the happiness of a trashcan.

On the fifteenth day, I was able to walk without limping.

Day after day, my list of improvements increased. The small wounds that normally stay open for weeks and infect easily as a result of the salty and humid environment on a boat healed perfectly in just a few days.

Since I started eating instinctively, despite the salty environment that comes with my lifestyle, the scarring process took only twelve to twenty-four hours. In only three days, the scab was gone. When I did not interfere, the healing process went without any pain.

At some point, I did revert to a traditional diet. But, twenty-four hours after a first spaghetti meal my brain remembered the pain. My headaches came back. Cooked meal after cooked meal I went down as I digested them. I tried to readjust to cooked food . . .

After eating cooked food for five days, on the morning of the sixth day, I woke up with my left foot paralyzed. Can it be clearer than that? This wasn't just another digestive problem. I had no choice and I stopped everything before another more violent crisis occurred.

Now I know that this way of eating doesn't change people. I believed it before, but didn't have enough distance for an objective judgment. Who I am today I already was before; it only cleaned the machine. And no matter the length of the path, no matter the effort I would have to put into it, I was ready to pay the price and go all the way, all the way to the core of myself. I moved on with a vague idea of the biological logic of happiness and most of all the certitude of not being born to suffer.

I recovered seventy percent of the sight in my left eye in two months.

I was in perfect health after only three months, but it took me almost a year to regain full psychological balance after what had happened.

I have been eating instinctively for fifteen years now.

On several occasions, I tried to revert back to a traditional diet, but my former symptoms always reappeared. Today, I live a normal life, and consider myself in a process of active remission as opposed to spontaneous remission characteristic in this type of disease.

Genefit Nutrition is a medical and social revolution, but would need more medical and public acceptance to make its long-term application easier.

Dominique G.

NAME: Roseline
YEAR OF BIRTH: 1941

My rheumatoid arthritis began in 1982, affecting my wrists with increasing stiffness, redness, pain, and inflammation, spreading to my knees, shoulders, and elbows. Anti-inflammatory treatment began in 1984, but was halted because of gastrointestinal side effects. I turned to naturopathy, with a diet of eggs, vegetables, limited fruit, and rice, for nine months. I then reverted to a "normal" diet for two months, which caused my symptoms to explode! I became paralyzed.

I began to eat instinctively in May 1985, at home, with a limited choice of fruits and vegetables. By the third day, I had developed a high fever and articulations were blocked (there was no elimination of toxins). When I began correct practice at the European Center near Paris, all my pain was gone in three weeks.

Today, I am extremely active and in good health. I can now hike eight kilometers or more.

My rheumatoid arthritis regressed almost completely in less than nine months.

Roseline

TWENTY

Food and Weight Management

LOSING WEIGHT under Genefit Nutritional eating conditions is automatic and effortless. As the immune system gets out of tolerance, it will do whatever is needed to restore the body's integrity. The body will then progressively regain its ideal weight. It is not unusual to see people lose from half a pound to one pound a day when eating by instinct. Not only is weight lost quickly, but it is also lost safely, because it is guided by your instinct. The rate will not exceed the limit your body can handle. The nutritional instinct expresses itself through pleasure, so that losing weight occurs without the frustations experienced with other diets. As a result, you won't have as much difficulty maintaining the diet as you would with other weight management approaches, which are based on food exclusions and food restrictions. Genefit Nutrition is probably the only way of eating where the maxim *the more you eat, the more you will lose* can be applied. It is unusual, but eating more can cause faster weight loss as a result of faster detoxination. Of course, all this will only happen if you need to lose weight. Otherwise, after a little weight loss resulting from the first detoxination waves, you will quickly stabilize at your ideal weight.

When food is chosen by instinct, it is not all about weight loss. While you lose unnecessary pounds, your instinct will choose foods that permit profound regeneration work that needs to be achieved.

Except for species that naturally put on fat to survive long and cold winters, obesity does not exist in the wild, even for animals that have easy access to food. It would be dangerous for any animal to be unable to move fast enough to escape a predator. Since obesity is the direct consequence of an unnatural diet, the return to a truly natural way of eating is the most adequate approach to correct it. In a truly natural food environment, when food is selected by instinct, overeating and obesity are virtually impossible. Nutrition achieves its real purpose, which is to nourish and maintain the body, instead of overloading it with unnecessary food molecules and empty calories.

TWENTY-ONE

Food and Cardiovascular Diseases

IF PROOF IS NEEDED for the accumulation of abnormal substances in the body, cardiovascular diseases are the most flagrant demonstration. Obviously, the body itself does not produce fat substances obstructing the arteries. They come from the food we eat, and more specifically, from denatured food. Unless there is a genetic problem, cardiovascular diseases do not exist in wild animals that have access to an optimal food supply; this is not only because of the large amount of exercise they get, but also because of the absence of accumulation of abnormal substances in their bodies. In addition, the very precise, instinctive food intake regulation mechanism protects them from overeating, as well as dietary imbalances, at all times. With unprocessed food, when digestive processes occur the way they are supposed to, there is nothing the body can or will accumulate that might harm it.

"Heating oils to deep-frying temperatures alters fatty acids chemically, which forms new chemical compounds, NCCs. . . . On analysis, the chemical structure of those compounds discloses them to be potentially toxic." It is as yet unclear whether those compounds can percolate through the bowel wall into lymph and subsequently into the bloodstream. To ascertain this, rats that had developed a fistula in their ribcage lymph duct were fed either heated soybean oil, incorporating a complex blend of new chemical compounds (NCCs), or a clearly structured purified NCC. Subsequently sampled and analyzed. "The results showed that 53 percent of the overall intake of oxidized monomer was recovered from the lymph in the ensuing 48 hours." Some rats were also parenterally tube-fed a cyclic acid (fatty acids having coupled as simple cycles) containing a cyclohexenic compound. Frying oil contains approximately 0.2 percent of such heat-released cyclic acids. "With this kind of dietary supplement, our results have shown that 95 percent of the cyclohexenic compound intake may be traced in the lymph" (N. Combe, M.J.Constantin, B. Entressangles, "How oxidative by-products released from heating oils makes its way into the lymph," *Journal of Nutrition and Diet*, Sept 1982, pp. 139-141).

Cardiovascular diseases are the number-one source of mortality, with 700,000 people dying each year in the U.S. alone. Cardiovascular diseases never appeared under Genefit Nutrition eating conditions. It seems that only a little wisdom and correct practice could bring those alarming numbers to zero, but for this to happen, a radical change of dietary habits is needed — a change far more demanding than taking medicine's "wonder pills."

TWENTY-TWO

Food and Diabetes

DIABETES IS THE NAME of a dysfunction of sugar metabolism that is widely misunderstood. It gradually leads to degeneration of the entire body, and normally never heals by itself. Medical treatment cannot cure it. It can only control it to some extent. The price of treatment can be high, since the drugs (in particular, insulin) give rise to other symptoms, which are also difficult to treat successfully. One of the most critical side effects of the treatment is loss of sight.

"Because of evidence that cow's milk intake can trigger diabetes in rodents, a study of diabetic children showed that antibodies to bovine serum albumin and a 17-amino-acid bovine serum albumin peptide (ABBOS). These antibodies would bind to a pancreatic beta-cell surface antigen.

This study showed that diabetic patients had high serum concentrations of anti-BSA antibodies (IgA and IgG). The presence of antibody (which means presence of antigen-specific B-cells) may signal the concomitant presence of antigen-specific cytotoxic T-lymphocytes, although these have not yet been demonstrated. The researchers suggest that . . . "relevant clones (of lymphocytes) are continuously transferred from immature IgM-expressing B-cell compartments to pools of IgG-secreting or IgA secreting cells." They go on to describe "a slow, inefficient process, consistent with the fact that clinical disease develops in only about 5 to 6 percent of hosts with the relevant genetic predisposition."

The diabetes model of food-antigen triggered disease is a potentially important immunological model of many unsolved diseases, which appear to be "autoimmune." A long-term, inefficient pathogenesis, which may produce target-organ damage, especially if the antigen is provided by a common food and intake continues over many years. Alternative explanations suggest that beta cells are attacked by cytotoxic T-cells after they have been infected by a virus, or by T-cells originally targeted on other cells infected by virus whose cell-surface antigens happen to resemble beta cell antigens.

An Australian study of children who developed diabetes found that children given cow's milk formula in the first three months were 52 percent more likely to develop diabetes than those not fed cow's milk. Breast-fed infants had a 34 percent lower incidence of diabetes than formula fed infants (Alpha Nutrition Health Education Series, Children's Center. *Cow's Milk Allergy in Children*).

Past observations give us an indication of the potential value of Genefit Nutrition in at least halting the progress of this disease, if not curing it. As with other maladies, the occurrence of diabetes demonstrates that denatured food damages the bodily functions of the person who eats it. Genefit Nutrition points to a path neither diabetics nor medical research can afford to neglect. For every diabetic known to have tried it, Genefit Nutrition rapidly reduced insulin dependency by at least fifty percent — and usually more. In theory at least, if this method of nutrition were adopted from the onset of the disease, it might well enable new diabetics to avoid becoming dependent on insulin altogether.

NAME: Genevieve D.
YEAR OF BIRTH: 1952

I have been diabetic for nearly seventeen years, using three injections of insulin daily for a total of forty units. I was able to reduce this dosage rapidly by a quarter and then by half. I did have an unpleasant period of detoxination, with glycemia over 2.50 g., but for the past fifteen days my need for insulin has been only ten units, my glycemia is often nearly normal, there is no longer any sugar in my urine, and acetone appears rarely or only as a trace.

Concerning my retinopathy, I had been seeing an ophthalmologist every three to six months, and at my last consultation I was told that "the inner eye is getting well." I was told to stop taking the two sorts of pills I had been using for seven years for my blood circulation because they were no longer needed, and the next appointment has been set for a year from now.

I also had a necrosed thyroid nodule that appeared six months after beginning treatment for a hyperthyroid condition that started three years ago. From the last echograph, it appeared that the necrosed tissues had all but completely disappeared!

Now, I feel really good. I have become much calmer and patient in my professional life. My cellulite has disappeared, something I had never been able to get rid of. I have no more digestive problems, no more colitis, no more intestinal gas. My diabetes specialist has witnessed all these improvements, but says not enough time has passed to make a real judgment. Clearly, the disappearance of the necrosed tissues of the nodule is unexplainable; in the 400 cases he knows of, nothing similar has ever been observed, even with hormone treatment. Nevertheless, he advised me to "not eat too much fruit." But I continue to trust my instinct!

Genevieve D.

TWENTY-THREE

Food and Viruses

LOUIS PASTEUR was the first to use the term "virus" to describe the pathogenic effect of bacteria that he had discovered under a microscope. At the beginning of the twentieth century, lenses with an increasingly high resolution, together with high-powered centrifugation, X-ray diffraction, and electrophoresis, helped prove the existence of minute particles, infective and indefinitely reproducible, though bereft of independent vitality. They reproduce themselves, but don't resemble our own cell structure, as bacteria do. They are impervious to antibiotics.

More recently, the advent of molecular biology and electronic microscopes has made it possible to specify and visualize accurately the structures of many viruses, as well as their reproduction and behavior. This investigation has lifted the veil of mystery those infinitesimal beings were so long shrouded in, determining the causation of many ailments and diseases, including those responsible for the tragedies of past diseases such as smallpox and poliomyelitis, and, in this day and age, AIDS. This knowledge affords us the hope of finding the effective protective strategies, whether they are

1. preventive, that is, working directly on the immune system through inoculation, or
2. curative, directly inhibiting viral activity within the molecules by means of drugs.

However, the enduring failure of these methods in the management of most viral diseases, in spite of the existing technological approach, leads us to ask a number of questions. The basis of reasoning that underlies present-day research has, in fact, been handed down from an era when man had hardly disentangled himself from superstitions connected to fear of contamination and horrendous epidemics. The manner in which past medicine depicted viruses — which were unquestioningly regarded as pathogenic, i.e., intrinsically harmful agents — is not inevitably the only one. Currently, illness is often seen to result from an imbalance between the host and the attacker, attributing more importance to factors liable to weaken body immunity resistance. A further step would involve studying the real meaning of viral activity, apart from any emotional bias. Put another way: Are viruses inherently "bad" in all cases?

In the classical model of viral phenomena, viruses are generally considered to be pathogenic agents, lacking any real life and living off the being they infect. Viruses are little more than a shell containing DNA or RNA, which they inject into a host cell after landing upon its surface. The viral particle fastens onto the membrane of a cell and sequences its DNA or RNA, subverting cellular genetics to viral reproduction. The new virions ("baby" viruses) spread through the bloodstream and lymph system and contaminate other cells. The immune system of the host reacts, more or less successfully, by releasing antibodies that put a halt to the process. This occurs belatedly and explains the varying shades of seriousness in regards to the symptoms observable in different people.

According to the classic view, the ultimate aim of the viral process is to ensure that the virus replicates and endures. The parasitic virus endures at the expense of a living being, which implies that the latter must survive, and does so within limits that strike a balance between the toxicity of the virus and the immunity of a species.

The genetic nucleotide sequences for a large number of viruses are now known, as well as the structure of their capsule and the type of antigen that enables identification by the host immune system. Sizeable sections of such sequences are identical in the virus and in the infected host. This kinship, which is required for the virus to subvert cell genetics, can hardly be accounted for by chance, since the likelihood of a suitably matched nucleotide mapping is virtually nil.

After a viral invasion, and in spite of defense mechanisms being marshaled, genetic viral data remain within the cell, either as inactivated viral particles or integrated into the cell genome. Such a feature explains the involvement of viruses in the evolution of species.

Viral invasion triggers a response from the immune system through a number of symptoms: exhaustion, high temperature, swelling, phlegm, rashes, and so on. Further, in respiratory tract diseases, the viral process commonly co-occurs with an increase in pathogenic bacteria numbers. In the normal course of events, this proliferation is halted, for example, in the common cold, through bacteriostasis of nasal mucus. But this balance seems broken by the action of the virus. Likewise, viral pneumonia can result in bacterial overinfection and in various complications. Practitioners employ antibiotic therapy, even though it isn't effective against the viral process proper. When there are no complications, viral disease spontaneously converges towards cure. In some cases, it can carry consequences, such as posthepatic cirrhosis, and can even result in death.

The classical methods of struggle against viral disease are prophylactics, vaccination, rest, diet, refraining from drinking and smoking, vitamin therapy, and antibiotics, in order to avoid bacterial complications. More recently, various molecules blocking the mechanisms of viral multiplication or antivirals (like AZT) were used, with results that were not always conclusive. In a general way, one can say that there is no really satisfactory treatment against viral disease.

There are, of course, a great many viruses in the natural world that cause no apparent harm. In many cases, viral diseases run a latent course and viral data can indeed remain in contaminated cells over long periods of time, without causing any particular symptoms. Anyone so infected is traditionally called, somewhat contradictorily, a "healthy (silent) carrier." With respect to most viruses, that state describes the vast majority of individuals. In a substantial number of cases, viral illness occurs in a frustrated, and thus asymptomatic, way (this includes ninety-nine percent of infections of the polio virus).

A number of viral infections arise, more often than not, in an asymptomatic way. Concerning poliomyelitis, for instance, serological surveys in contaminating circumstances have shown that the nervous system is only affected in a marginal number of contaminated individuals. In children, first contact with the oral herpes virus typically occurs latently, and in adults, sequels are rare, with most individuals being silent carriers. Many latent forms of the hepatitis virus also exist. Mild forms commonly find an outlet in the full recovery of hepatocytes. The structure of the liver cells fully returns to normal, because the reticulum holds up well throughout the course of the disease. Likewise, the Epstein-Barr virus goes undetected in most cases, except when blood tests and serum tests are performed. Although it occurs in the majority of African children, it only sets up Burkitt's sarcoma in one case out of 10,000, presumably aided by various cofactors. Whenever the virus causes mononucleosis, the disease normally remains minor. Rabies does show telltale symptoms in some people, though not in others. It is still not known why the disease runs different courses in different cases.

The same phenomenon is true for animals. Bird influenza occurs in domestic ducks and quails, causing coughing, sneezing, and swelling around the bill—which developments bring about a fairly high death rate—whereas the flu remains benign or latent in other species, both wild and domestic. Pig influenza carries a serious, and possibly lethal, prognosis for piglets contaminated by the sow. It occurs in pigs from different areas, and it very rarely shows up clinically. Many epidemiologists believe that most viruses are very widespread throughout every species, including humans, but only show signs of disease occasionally, due to the effect of little-understood causative cofactors.

The fact that the number of latent forms and silent carriers of a disease turns out to be greater than that of serious forms can only encourage us to reassess traditional models of reasoning. It is quite possible that an asymptomatic mode of viral invasion is quite normal, whereas disease-causing forms may merely be the result of random factors, attributable to further pathogenic factors.

By analogy, imagine rockets being launched to put satellites into orbit. If launching fails once in every ten attempts, it might appear that the aim of the game was to blow up the satellites, and that the operation failed on nine occasions. A potential onlooker might be unaware of what actual intent lies behind observable facts. Furthermore, if he doesn't know that satellites do have a purpose, he might think it useful to step in and blow the satellite to smithereens with basic explosives, rather than try to help make the launch a success. Viruses, like satellites, may be of benefit to us in most cases. Since our attention is rarely drawn to viruses, except in cases where they are being attacked by the immune system, it is easy to overlook the possibility that they are beneficial.

Most viruses severely disrupt health in only about one percent of cases. Obviously, one can only think them awesome if their sole purpose is to cause mayhem. However, if our contention were substantiated, and viral processes are indeed endowed with purpose, not excluding a possible investigation of why and when they go wrong and accidentally turn dangerous, this would markedly alter the course of research. If broadminded researchers investigated the hypothesis that viruses are ordinarily symbiotic, and only occasionally become dangerous, better understanding of viral phenomena and valuable applications to therapy could result.

As for AIDS, the virus known as HIV was initially believed to be nefarious in all cases. Significantly, some researchers came to the conclusion, only ten years after the virus was discovered, that the pathogenic impact of that retrovirus was owing more to particular cofactors than to its inherent features. Considering the dismal failure of the prevention and courses of treatment implemented and, further, considering how critical the situation has become, it is worth leaving no stone unturned. Just as whenever a theory gets caught in deadlock or proves powerless, so the very basis of medical reasoning must be recast in the light of new evidence, especially when facts are supported by fresh experiments.

It has been noted that under conditions of Genefit Nutrition, almost all viral diseases develop in an either mild or asymptomatic way. Viral invasion and a swarm of viral particles appear to occur, however, in conditions not unlike typical ones. It is generally admitted that the spread of viral infection depends on the overall state of the patient, but the factors characterizing this state have not yet been clearly established. Under Genefit Nutrition eating conditions, however, even when the disease remained silent, contaminated individuals presented with typical symptoms only hours after a traditional meal of processed food, i.e., as soon as abnormal molecules, which seem to be the cause of the symptoms, had entered bodily fluids. Given the prerequisite of truly natural eating conditions, in line with the genetic needs of the body, the absence or alleviation of symptoms denoting viral diseases should, by rights, warrant rethinking the very concept of viral diseases as it has so far been defined.

A preliminary interpretation would be conceding quite simply that eating a natural diet is more protective against a viral onslaught. But one could view the problem in an entirely different light and no longer consider the virus as a pathogenic agent itself, but rather consider pathogenic symptoms that ought to be investigated in other factors, which might prove the genetic unsuitability of unnatural and processed foods.

More to the point, it would be worth considering whether viruses, which are so common in the natural world, are not endowed with a biological assignment whose teleological meaning is a closed book to contemporary medicine — at any rate, when it comes to human beings. What could we learn from how viruses affect other species in the wild?

Under conditions of Genefit Nutrition, a patient with virtually any viral disease presents with discharges, such as phlegm, perspiration, rashes, diarrhea, overcharged urine, oversecretion of skin oils, specific body odors, and so on. In view of such common experiential evidence, along with current data provided by enzymology, molecular biology, virology, and immunology, it could be concluded that besides coding for conditions necessary for the replication of viral particles, DNA or viral RNA also sequences protein synthesis, which enables the body to clear given abnormal molecules alien to normal metabolism that might have built up within the cells.

Admittedly, retroviruses are only endowed with a highly restricted genome and only synthesize a minute number of differing proteins, whose functions have, in most cases, already been documented. However, a given protein may, nonetheless, demonstrate a dual function, the first one pertaining to the replication of the virus, and the second involving an as yet little understood process of serviceability to the cell. Biology has been known to have such surprises in store for us: many organs exhibit manifold functions, and some genes may be decoded by staggering a nucleotide, thus giving rise to two different, and yet functional, proteins, and so on. Not inconceivably, a viral protein could, for instance, be construed both to suppress viral replication and also to bind with a given group of abnormal molecules in order to ferry them out of the cell. In such a way, viral swarm would be associated with a concentration of abnormal molecules, accounting for the self-regulatory process.

In the light of the foregoing discussion, viruses, or at any rate, some viruses, might be viewed as complementing the immune system as traditionally described. The system ensures the synthesis of antibodies commissioned to clear antigens within bodily fluids, whereas viruses would, hypothetically, be agents for some kind of intracellular immune function, empowering them for the upkeep of law and order inside cells.

In other words, the virus provides the cell with whatever genetic material it requires to identify and clear molecules it cannot control through its own genetic code. Such molecules, alien to normal breakdown, are taken up by the body from various environmental sources, including processed foods harboring (or consisting of) molecules the body is not genetically equipped to deal with. The symptoms that show up during viral development result primarily from the difficulty a body has in clearing those molecules, rather than from waging a struggle against the actual virus.

In this new model, the viruses and bacteria involved in the genesis of most so-called infectious diseases are regarded as vectors and partners in genetically encoded symbiotic processes, which help the body clear molecules alien to organic functions inside actual cells. These processes indicate disease when an overload of abnormal molecules occurs in body fluids — this being bound up with inadequate dietary habits — since the workings of human metabolism are unable to handle changes in such culinary practices that have been with us since the beginning of food processing, and increasingly so in more recent times.

It may be suggested that the large-scale use of antibiotic courses of treatment and inoculations — inasmuch as they have inhibited the processes described above — may have prompted the advent of degenerative and autoimmune diseases, as well as carcinomatosis, subsequent to the build-up of abnormal molecules, whether antigenic or life-unfriendly, inside the body. It could be the abnormal molecules, rather than the viruses, that disrupt immunological and biological functions required for the maintenance of health.

As for HIV, virtually anyone infected was thought to experience serious symptoms. Experiences of people using Genefit Nutrition seem to contradict such arguments. In recent years, the same or similar retroviruses have been discovered in many wild animals that did not appear sick in any way. Some researchers concluded that the virus was not actually disease causing, rather that as yet unknown cofactors were at work.

In the Genefit Nutritional view, those cofactors could well be abnormal molecules that have built up much more in humans than in wild animals, and that the virus is commissioned to clear away. The viral processes devised to sequence the clearance of abnormal molecules in an initially silent way are now being overrun: the surfeit of target molecules is believed to disrupt the regulatory processes that ensured its proper functioning, and, most notably, bring out opportunistic infections that are dangerous due to the over-expansion of bacteria relevant to the clearing of the same molecules. Why, therefore, should it be that the HIV retrovirus, which may have been part of man's low-profile genetic legacy, as is the case for animals, should have reared its head out of cell nuclei to trigger a serious epidemic? Indisputably, the causes instrumental in this phenomenon include sweeping dietary changes over the last few decades, especially in Third World countries where Western dietary habits have spread like wildfire, as have fresh sources of contamination. Having been sparked off, viral replication could not but spread like wildfire, too: the most highly contagious viral particles and those that affect mucous membranes the most are the fastest spreading.

What is more, organisms that no longer harbored the virus, or in whom it had been thoroughly mothballed, have had ample time to collect a high amount of target molecules. This accounts for the uncanny aggressiveness of the viral process, further magnified by the daily intake of foods that are vectors for molecules from the same groups.

TWENTY-FOUR

Food and the Practice of Medicine

Patrick Fontanaud, M.D.
Physician with specialization in homeopathy

The first time I heard about Genefit Nutrition was in 1983, during a lecture in the city of Bordeaux, France.

Impressed by the concept, I soon after attended a seminar.

Genefit Nutrition strongly challenged my certitudes and it took me a few weeks to "digest" this new and revolutionary approach to eating. But in analyzing the facts, critiquing the theoretical foundation, and being as objective as possible, I realized there are only very few points that are really questionable.

As a physician, I believe that this way of eating matches the physiology of human beings and should be applied as such. From knowing and applying this method of eating, I observed rheumatic pain disappear, tiredness subside, unnecessary pounds melt away, allergies and psoriasis fade, etc.

Genefit Nutrition should be used as a therapeutic instrument to improve common pathologies. Personally, Genefit Nutrition has changed my life, but I am also aware of the obstacles for its application. It is, nonetheless, possible to recover or maintain health in applying Genefit Nutrition over limited periods of time and adapted to the lifestyle of each of us.

Patrick Fontanaud

Dr. Jean Seignalet
Immunology Laboratory
Hospital St. Eloi
Montpellier, France

After attending a lecture on the theoretical foundations of Genefit Nutrition, Dr. Jean Seignalet decided to undertake a large-scale experiment with a diet he prescribed to an impressive number of patients. The following are the results of his dietary method, which totally excluded wheat and its by-products, milk and dairy products, and included as much raw food as possible[1]:

Diseases	# of cases	Total remissions	Improvements 90%	Improvements 50%	Failures	Success rate*
Rheumatoid Arthritis	200	83	66	11	40	80%
Ankylosing Spondylitis	100	63	33		4	96%
Psoriatic Arthritis	25	10	8	6	1	96%
Pseudo Polyarthritis Rhizomélic	13	10	3			100%
Juvenile Arthritis	7	5		1	1	
ACJ Polyarticular	4		2		2	
ACJ Oligoarticulary	1				1	
Palindromic Rheumatism	4	3			1	
Inflammatory Rheumatism	8	6		2		
Gougerot-Sjögren	65	11	10	28	16	75%
Systemic Lupus Erythematosus	13	6	3	4		100%
Scleroderma	10		10			100%
Dermatomyositis	1		1			
Mixed Connectivity	3		2		1	
Lupus	5	1	2	2		
Fascite of Schulman	1		1			
Hashimoto's Disease	8			8		
Multiple Sclerosis	33	9	15	8	1	97%
Lapeyronie's Disease	4	2	2			
Myasthenia	1			1		
Idiopathic Thromb. Purpura	2				2	

Diseases	# of cases	Total remissions	Improvements 90%	50%	Failures	Success rate*
Chronic Active Hepatitis	1	1				
Anterior Uveitis	10	8	2			100%
Guillain Barré	1		1			
Peripheral Neuropathy	6		1	4	1	
Primary Biliary Cirrhosis	1		1			
Wegener's granulomatosis	2		1	1		
Allergic Granulomatous Angiitis	1			1		
Fibromyalgia	41	25	8	7	1	97%
Tendinitis	10	6	2		2	80%
Arthrosis	26	9	10	7		100%
Osteoporosis	20	No further progression of the disease in 50 percent of the cases				
Gout	2	2				
Chondrocalcinosis	2		2			
Migraines	40	26	8		6	85%
Manic Depressive Psychosis	1		1			
Depression	16	12	3		1	93%
Parkinson's Disease	6		2	2	2	
Dystonia	1	1				
Type 1 Diabetes	14	11		3		100%
Hypoglycemia	4	4				
Hypercholesterolemia	66	Reduction of cholesterol by 30 percent				
Spasmosphilia	26	20	3	1	2	92%
Overweight	100	30	25	25	20	80%
Aplasie Medullaire	2	1			1	
Leucemia	8	5	1		2	
Irritable Bowel Syndrome	220	215			5	98%
Colitis	3	2			1	
Ulcerative Colitis	8			3	5	
Crohn's Disease	40	33	2	5		100%
Acne	40	35	5			100%
Atopic Eczema	11	6	4	1		100%
Urticaria	15	14			1	93%
Angeitis	4	2			2	

Diseases	# of cases	Total remissions	Improvements 90%	Improvements 50%	Failures	Success rate*
Psoriasis	53	33	4	4	12	77%
Bronchitis	8	8				
Asthma	51	46		3	2	96%
Infections ORL Chronic	100	80			20	80%
Chronic Sinusitis	6	6				
Hay Fever	35	30	2	3		100%
Simple Chronic Rhinitis	18	18				100%
Allergic Conjunctivitis	12	12				100%
Angioneurotic Edema	13	13				100%
Aphtosis	12	6	4	2		100%
Histiocytosis	1		1			
Urticaria Pigmentosa	1		1			
Chronic Fatigue Syndrome	11	2		7	2	82%

*Success rates include remission and improvements down to 50 percent.
1. "Nutrition or the Third Medicine." Dr. Jean Seignalet—edition Francois-Xavier de Guilbert, Paris.

Jean Devernois de Bonnefon, M.D.
Former Clinic Chief, Salpetriere Hospital, Paris
Medical Expert at the Paris Court of Appeals

What I Think About Genefit Nutrition

1. Unlike philosophical or naturopathic diets, all of which are exclusion diets based on an idea (e.g., vegetarianism, vegan, macrobiotics, etc.), Genefit Nutrition does not appear dangerous to me in that it allows for all foods except milk: glucides, lipids, animal or vegetable proteins, and even the use of as many as possible in all their natural variety. It is safe on condition that it is correctly applied, through the use of olfactory and gustatory senses once they have been reawakened.

2. Genefit Nutrition is not medicine since it makes no use of diagnoses, chemical products, or technical expedients. On the contrary, it

counters alimentary artifice, which we are beginning to see is endangering our health and is a cause of disease.

It is not even a diet, since no dietary prescription exists. In effect, it is the individual who chooses. It is his body that does so, not his mind. And his body probably knows better than any computer what it needs, and what is most useful in an ongoing and specific way. Genefit Nutrition is in no way contrary to, or incompatible with, medicine. The usefulness and necessity of medicine is preserved in fighting symptoms and illnesses, while Genefit Nutrition consolidates the terrain by way of its nourishment. In my view, Genefit Nutrition can only reinforce tolerance to, and the effectiveness of, chemical medicine. Medicine and Genefit Nutrition are therefore complementary. And this is true even in cases of severe illness, where it is appropriate to employ as many weapons as possible.

3. In practical terms, insofar as I have been able to see and experiment, Genefit Nutrition is surprisingly effective as concerns the improvement of well persons, and a return to health for sick ones.

4. On theoretical grounds, Genefit Nutrition addresses three essential questions:

a. The disturbing problem of the accelerating denaturation of our food
b. The problem of the role of our nutritional instinct, completely ignored by our teaching hospitals
c. The question of our genetic and enzymatic adaptation to our nutrition.

In summary, this method of nutrition, on condition that it is correctly applied, is the best dietetic approach I know of, and I feel that its application in the form of an intensive cure can be extremely useful for our health.

Jean Devernois de Bonnefon, M.D.

PART FIVE

Genefit Nutrition: Past, Present, and Future

TWENTY FIVE

Testimonials

NAME: Guenther B.
YEAR OF BIRTH: 1960

How a little book can change your life . . .

It happened under the sunshade on the Adriatic Sea in the summer of 1992. Destiny shuffled a book in my hands about eating instinctively and all of a sudden it crossed my mind: "This is the most important discovery of mankind since the invention of writing!" There was no doubt: I was on the most important path of my life.

I wanted to find out the truth about all this and decided to try it out myself. It certainly wouldn't do any harm if I ate fruit and vegetables for a month. I felt good, I lost weight, and life was better than ever before. So I extended the experiment to three months and then to a year. Now it has been nine years giving marvelous results!

Within a year I lost more than 27 kg (60 pounds) of bodyweight, especially after learning about the importance of eating truly natural foods of Purefood quality. After I reached 60 kg I started gaining some weight again and then I stabilized. I enjoyed nuts, macadamia and later peanuts, seasonal fruits and vegetables! I enjoy eating as much as I want. My weight is steady at around 68kg (I'm 5' 9" tall).

For nine years, I have never had any need for medication and I never skipped a day of work for sickness. I have gained a lot of energy. I have built up my own consulting company and worked hard for the last five years with almost no holidays! All this stress did not have any repercussions for my health, and my venture gave me great satisfaction.

My new lifestyle is all based on believing in nature! When I follow this natural way of life I feel that I am growing into an extraordinary spiritual existence. At this time I really don't know where this road will lead me, but it feels like heaven.

Guenther B.

NAME: Anne B.
YEAR OF BIRTH: 1944

Thinking back to the time before Genefit Nutrition, I still remember very clearly when I started feeling old. It was at the age of thirty-five, when little discomforts became chronic instead of disappearing quickly: migraine-like headaches, frequent infections, eczema especially in my face, digestive difficulties, swollen mucous membranes, sensitive bladder, and ringing in my ears before going to sleep. Generally I felt exhausted already when I got up in the morning.

At the age of forty-seven, I discovered a German book about instinctive eating. In order to improve my condition, I was ready to try whatever was available in the field of alternative approaches to nutrition. The content of the book was outstanding in comparison to other diet books that were mostly based on unfounded assumptions reinforced by a dogma. In addition, I was also glad to learn that Genefit Nutrition could have implications far beyond a simple diet

I decided to approach the new discovery slowly, starting out with fruits in the morning instead of bread following the concepts of *Fit for Life* by Harvey and Marilyn Diamond. The immediate results were surprising: I felt more awake and present.

While on a vacation with my mother, I left my husband at home alone and it was his turn to discover the book. After experimenting for six weeks on our own, we took an introduction seminar, and six months later a 21-day Genefit Nutrition retreat.

The twenty-one days of hundred- percent practice were enough to eliminate all the health issues I had been dealing with before. There was no more tiredness or exhaustion.

Ten years later, I am still applying many ideas of Genefit Nutrition, and eat eighty percent raw foods. I eat fruit for lunch and vegetables for dinner instinctively, adding some processed foods at night that I choose carefully. I feel fresh, awake, and agile in the morning with plenty of energy for the day. I can easily compete with people twenty years younger than I am, except of course those practicing Genefit Nutrition at a hundred percent.

As far as my health issues and signs of age are concerned, they stay away as long as I don't eat too much processed food. Whenever they return in a light form, I interpret them as a warning sign encouraging me to be stricter about what I eat and usually they disappear quickly. I am now so used to feeling so perfectly well, that I interpret even a slight sweat at night or a bad taste in my mouth in the morning as abnormal. However, I have none of the health issues of others of my age.

On a psychological level, I enjoy more inner calm and peace, which I notice especially in high-stress situations. I feel more alive, more courage and trust, and more access to intuition. By seeing how Genefit Nutrition can be effective, I have found more confidence in the wisdom of my body and my psyche.

Anne B.

NAME: Francis D.
YEAR OF BIRTH: 1946

My health during adolescence was fragile. In 1964, when I was eighteen years old, I obtained health improvements after changing to a so-called "naturopathic diet" without refined sugar, white flower, coffee, or chemical additives. But I still caught serious colds lasting four to five months a year.

In 1974, at age twenty-six, I contracted some kind of genital herpes (physicians didn't know exactly what it was, nor could they help). More problems, also difficult to diagnose, appeared again before I reached forty: thigh-skin reddening with pimples, tingling in the legs when I have been seated for a long time, serious lower back pain, and so on, every one of these problems worsening with time, as did the colds.

I started eating instinctively in January 1987. I noticed improvements right away. Almost all my health problems disappeared immediately. Only one problem didn't improve much, but it didn't get worse either: a cyst. My lower back pain disappeared 90 and 95 percent with less acute and shorter crises. My sleep is much better and bad dreams are a thing of the past.

Since the age of thirty-seven, I have taken no medicine. I have practiced instinctive eating for fifteen years, and have eaten no cooked food since.

Eating by instinct is a routine now, but it's also a great pleasure. By the way, pleasure is the main reason why I went on for so long with this way of eating. First, I started to experiment with the nutritional instinct for five days or so. Then I went on for a month, three months, a year, another year. . . . I might return to cooked food one day, maybe tomorrow or maybe ten years from now, I don't know. So I feel free, and not enclosed in a system for my whole life, which is very important psychologically.

I can consider myself lucky to have access to a lot of very good tropical fruits, meat, oysters, nuts, and other foodstuffs from local markets. Eggs are the only food still difficult to obtain, especially off season.

In my lifetime, I have traveled three times around the world, finding sufficient food almost everywhere — as long as I stayed not too far from the ocean.

The theory behind Genefit Nutrition is logical and simple, but the practice can be difficult in the beginning. As long as one considers it to be as an experiment of limited duration, one should be able to live with it without social and psychological problems. It is important not to limit the choice of foods for intellectual or cultural reasons and to always question the theoretical background, and so not consider it the ultimate truth.

Francis D.

NAME: *France M.*
YEAR OF BIRTH: 1952

I had been suffering from fibroids, which were diagnosed in December 1980, during the pregnancy with my first child. The symptoms took the form of long, painful, and abundant menstrual periods. I never had any treatment for it but the symptoms increased between 1980 and 1991 and disappeared about one and a half months after starting Genefit Nutrition.

I also had a bunch of other health issues such as hemorrhoids, osteoarthritis, and rheumatic pain. All these problems disappeared only one month after changing my diet.

My children, born in 1981, 1984, and 1985, had many health issues too (ear infections that needed drains for several years, pharyngitis and sinusitis that antibiotics could not eradicate, a continuous series of ENT diseases since birth).

My three children did not start eating everything unprocessed right away, but I decided to exclude milk, dairy, and wheat products in December 1991. Their transition to Genefit Nutrition was progressive. My son was very nervous and aggressive at home and absentminded at school. He had trouble sleeping. After changing their diet, they all lost weight at first, but then their various problems disappeared. Their school results increased impressively. Now, they are sixteen, eighteen, and twenty years old, and they are magnificent young people, healthy in their bodies and minds. They have all decided to keep eating instinctively.

France M.

TWENTY-SIX

Genefit Nutrition:
A Vision of the Future

IN THE PREVIOUS CHAPTERS, we have focused mainly on the medical and therapeutic aspects of Genefit Nutrition. We have done so in response to the ever-growing health issues faced by our societies. Nonetheless, we chose to end this book on a different note. We would like to see this last chapter describing a vision — a vision of what the world would be if the principles of Genefit Nutrition were to be applied globally. Of course, such a thing might not happen soon enough for us to witness, but it might be of some interest to explore all its implications.

First of all, it is important to point out that Genefit Nutrition is *not* antithetical to culture. In the past, the nurture/nature (acquired/innate) conflict has been excessively emphasized. Once we acknowledge that our cultural context partially originates from unnatural eating conditions, and that human instinctive behavior becomes detrimentally altered by the same eating conditions, we can easily understand why. Doesn't our evolutionary history tell us that processing is, to a great extent, responsible for the dichotomy? Without it, the view of a conflict between nature and nurture would almost certainly never have existed in the first place. Now might be the time to study in more depth how nurture can build upon nature. If Genefit Nutrition is, by essence, not opposed to culture and tradition, it nonetheless would change the course of cultural development, in the sense that education would, more than ever, take into consideration primary laws of nature and related genetic requirements.

If a majority of people ate by Genefit Nutrition principles, a new eating culture would see the light. For instance, Japanese, Indian, or Thai restaurants and American fast-food chains would probably be replaced by gourmet places where we could find rare fruits and other unprocessed foods native to those countries. The earth's rainforests would be subject to "gastronomical" inquiries, in addition to pharmaceutical ones, because of the immense variety of unknown fruits and plants they contain. Many plants and fruits available in the wild still do not have a name in a botanical sense. Thousands of new tastes and amazing flavors could thus be reintroduced into our food palette with clear benefits for our health and the environment. Many botanically classified fruits have been considered commercially uninteresting, because overloads and chemical imbalance produced by cooked foods make it impossible to eat or enjoy them. Once we break the boundaries held up by the commercial considerations of our dependence on processed food, the diversity of unprocessed foods available in nature seems limitless.

Furthermore, endless cornfields, wheat fields, and soybean fields would soon find themselves replaced by beautiful orchards, with hundreds or even thousands of different varieties of fruits trees. Since Genefit Nutrition reaches its full dimension with the widest diversity of food possible, it would be the end of the commercial monoculture so destructive to the environment. Instead of destroying primary forests to satisfy our eating needs, we could improve existing natural landscapes by adding fruit trees and other edible plants upon which we and other animals could feed. Supported by this view, permaculture has become increasingly popular today. The nutritional efficiency of an acre cultivated according to the principles of permaculture is up to ten times higher when compared to the same surface cultivated along the guidelines of monoculture. The amount of food so produced largely exceeds the amount any cornfield or soybean field could ever produce, with much less work. The positive impact on the environment would be tremendous. Monoculture, because of the ecological imbalance it creates, attracts parasites and diseases. As a result, pesticides become necessary to avoid losses. There are many ways to control parasite and insect development by balancing the existing ecosystem. In addition, many nonhybridized and nongrafted plants do well when it comes to parasites and diseases, especially when they are part of a diverse flora and fauna; by adjusting its natural balance, the recreated ecosystem can then expand, for the benefit of all the species involved. Nonhybridized plants reproduce by themselves and need little or no care. Wild plants survived long before humans learned how to plant a seed.

When fruit trees are mixed with nonfruit-producing trees, fertilizer and chemical soil balance is naturally provided. It is only when fruit trees are planted within an unnatural concentration that the soil becomes deprived of its nutrients. Fertilizers then become mandatory. A balanced ecosystem, built on a wide array of diverse plants and animals, needs very little work; it is self-perpetuating and self-sufficient. Today, still existing hunter-gatherer tribes spend an average of less than two hours a day to satisfy their nutritional needs, cooking and food preparation included. If we take cooking and other forms of processing away, those numbers can be brought to one hour at maximum. That leaves a lot of time for all the other activities we might want to do in our lives. With Genefit Nutrition, human beings, instead of being parasites to the environment, could contribute to its enrichment and be totally integrated into earth's ecosystem to become part of the whole once again.

In light of the foregoing, we can imagine that hunger would drastically drop not only in industrialized countries, but also in Third World countries — usually tropical or subtropical countries, where plant food grows relatively easily. In Africa, massive tree cutting still takes place in order to use wood for cooking purposes. Such practices strongly contribute to expand desertification. This process could be inverted and efforts could be made to plant and grow as many fruit trees as possible, and so eradicate not only Third World hunger, but also most of the catastrophic health problems those countries currently face.

Over time, Genefit Nutrition would spontaneously promote environmental consciousness. When food is eaten as nature provides it, each meal is a reminder of where food is actually coming from. A well-furnished Genefit Nutrition table is full of colors and shapes, an expression of nature's beauty, visually adding to the high level of eating pleasure

Genefit Nutrition provides. Holidays would match the beginnings of harvest seasons and give them a deeper meaning. Every time an intensely sought fruit comes in season, it would be an occasion for festivities.

Observations of the preventive and curative benefits of Genefit Nutrition have been more than conclusive. If more of a diversity of plants (especially wild plants from the rainforest that primates already use for self-medication) would be introduced in the eating palette of future generations, those benefits would probably continue to increase. Extrapolating on the observations we have been able to make, it might not be an exaggeration to state that three-quarters of the pathologies currently affecting Western civilizations would subside. Pain and suffering related to a disease would probably become exceptional rather than commonplace. Obesity would be an affliction of the past. A majority of the population would probably die a natural death, rather than die as a result of health problems. The amount of money currently spent on all kinds of medical treatments, as well as antidepressants, painkillers, and tranquilizers, would drastically drop, and could be reinvested in research, environmental projects, and many other similarly useful activities.

The behavioral and psychological changes observed with Genefit Nutrition are far from negligible. Because of the general relaxation of the nervous system, and a consequent decrease in aggressiveness, conflicts and problems could be faced with more equanimity. This is, of course, true for small everyday life problems as well as for large-scale political conflicts. With the increasingly easy access of weapons of mass destruction, the psychological balance of each individual on the planet becomes everyone's concern. When abnormal molecules, originating from food processing, hinder the brain's original way of functioning, they can only amplify already existing psychological problems. The absence of chemically induced emotions would probably help target the origin of the problems, instead of focusing exclusively on a remedy for their symptoms. In addition, Genefit Nutrition lowers anxieties, promotes individuality, boosts creativity, improves intuition, and spontaneously changes priorities in life. The unique state of mind produced by Genefit Nutrition clearly would alter the way people relate to each other, modify the way we look at the world, and help us equitably share the planet, despite our differences.

Of course, this remains, for now, only a vision — a dream. But let us remember that not so long ago, at the very beginning of the past century, the Wright brothers were convinced that one day man would fly. They dedicated their lives to building a machine they called a "flying-machine." Before its first public flight, the idea that such a machine might ever fly seemed, for many people, ridiculous, and its realization unfeasible. Similarly, some people envisioned that we would someday walk the surface of the moon. In 1865, one hundred and four years before the first man set foot on the moon, Jules Verne's novel *From the Earth to the Moon* was considered a fantastical story. However, during the entire time before the actual event, it was nothing but a fantastical story.

The power of the human mind to create is limitless. The happiness and well being of future generations depends on what we put our energy into. It depends on our priorities. Some of these priorities could undoubtedly change if we change the content of our daily meals.

Genefit Nutrition, LLC

GENEFIT NUTRITION is a California-based company dedicated to making the concepts of Genefit Nutrition available worldwide. It offers a wide range of educational services in the form of:

1. A COMPLETE GENEFIT NUTRITION TUTORIAL

Several decades of research condensed in one single tutorial. The informational equivalent of a ten hours real-life seminar — all you need for a perfect start on Genefit Nutrition. Thanks to our Online Tutorial, you can learn how to apply the principles of Genefit Nutrition at your own pace from the quietness of your home. The tutorial can be accessed at any time, anywhere in the world. For details please visit our web site at www.genefitnutrition.com.

a) Text Version includes:

- Diagrams
- Tables
- Meal Guide
- Articles

Paper edition, CD-Rom and online (56K, DSL, Cable). Available now at www.genefitnutrition.com!

b) Audio Version includes:

- 10 hours of audio recording
- Diagrams
- Tables
- Meal Guide
- Articles

Available Summer 2003 on CD and online (56K , DSL, Cable)

c) Multimedia Version includes:

- Audio sequences
- Video footage
- Animations
- Diagrams
- Tables
- Meal Guide
- Articles

Available Summer 2004 on DVD and online for high speed Internet access only (T1, DSL, Cable)

2. GENEFIT NUTRITION RETREATS

Our retreats are primarily about change. In addition to discovering a new way of eating, you will learn how to use Genefit Nutrition as a springboard to transform your life. Genefit Nutrition retreats are available in different locations, several times a year. Please call for details.

A 21-Day Retreat includes:

- All practical information to successfully apply Genefit Nutrition
- Workshops about the theoretical foundations of Genefit Nutrition
- Personal assistance during all meals
- Wide array of highest-quality, unprocessed foods
- Coaching and personal support during the entire 21-day cleanse
- Individual and group processing time
- After-program advice

3. ONE-ON-ONE COACHING SERVICES*

A complete coaching service includes:

- Individualized Genefit Nutrition coaching
- Complete in-home and on-location service with food delivery
- Assistance and guidance during each meal
- Wide array of highest-quality, unprocessed food supply
- 24/7 phone availability
- After-program advice

*Coaching services are available in the Hollywood–Los Angeles area. For all other nationwide or international locations, arrangements are possible. Please call for details.

4. IF YOU ARE A HEALTH PROFESSIONAL

With Genefit Nutrition, we certainly don't intend to offer an alternative to medical care. In most cases, Genefit Nutrition does not conflict with medical treatments. We believe that diverse opportunities should be available to every patient, especially those with serious conditions. Recovery can be facilitated if help comes from both sources: a truly natural diet and an appropriate treatment. A patient can only profit from a combined effort to reestablish the natural integrity of his body. As a health professional, you might want to recommend Genefit Nutrition to your patients. As we indicated, for Genefit Nutrition to work at a therapeutic level, it has to be practiced in a very precise manner. In response to this need, we offer educational programs specifically designed for health professionals about when and how to apply Genefit Nutrition in the most common diseases. Please contact us if you are interested in those programs.

For further questions about the above services, call us at:

GENEFIT NUTRITION, LLC
PHONE: 1-866-EATWISE
EMAIL: info@genefitnutrition.com
WEB: http://www.genefitnutrition.com

The Purefood Network

THE PUREFOOD NETWORK is a nonprofit organization that has been created to address the challenge of acquiring the food quality Genefit Nutrition requires. The company gave its name to a quality label and certifies growers and farmers who produce the highest quality unprocessed food. In order to make the application of Genefit Nutrition as convenient as possible. The Purefood Network offers:

1. A GENEFIT NUTRITION 21-DAY PACKAGE

It provides all you need to get started, including:

- A wide array of high-quality unprocessed foods
- The equivalent of a weekend introductory seminar in the form of a Beginner's Manual or a Multimedia CD-ROM

Boxes full of guaranteed unprocessed foods will be shipped every week to the address you provide — it can be your home address or a temporary vacation address. Currently, the Genefit Nutrition 21-day package is available in the U.S. only.

2. A YEARLY PUREFOOD MEMBERSHIP

A Purefood membership will give you access to the Purefood database, listing growers and farmers offering Genefit Nutrition–friendly foods online. Please call for details or visit Purefood online at http://www .the purefoodnetwork.com.

THE PUREFOOD NETWORK
PHONE: 1-866-EATPURE
EMAIL: info@thepurefoodnetwork.com
WEB: http://www.thepurefoodnetwork.com

The American Foundation for Genetic and Nutritional Anthropology

THE AMERICAN FOUNDATION for Genetic and Nutritional Anthropology is a nonprofit organization dedicated to the advancement of scientific research exploring the benefits of an instinctive pre-Paleolithic diet.

Probably because of its radically innovative nature, Genefit Nutrition grew up outside mainstream research pathways. We do not define ourselves as researchers as much as witnesses — people who have been able to observe unprecedented phenomena in themselves and others. Our goal is not to confront or compete with traditional research, but rather to share our experience and observations. In doing so, we hope to provide enough convincing information to raise the interest of institutional researchers. We would like to see the scientific community take over more and more the exploration of the hypothesis Genefit Nutrition is based on. Among all the people who have applied Genefit Nutrition over the past four decades, we count an impressive number of physiological and psychological improvements. Still, further research needs to be done to understand the mechanisms at work when switching to this way of eating. Hopefully, more studies will keep confirming what has been observed so far.

As a researcher, there are two ways you can help:

1. Join our research committee. The American Foundation for Genetic and Nutritional Anthropology offers memberships in its growing research committee. If this book had a major impact on you, and you feel Genefit Nutrition should be studied in more depth, you are invited to become a member. For more information about memberships, contact us at commitee@afgna.org.
2. Setup studies related to Genefit Nutrition yourself. You are welcome to contact us at research@afgna.org for questions or assistance.

IF YOU WOULD LIKE TO SUPPORT
GENEFIT NUTRITIONAL RESEARCH

For the advancement of research, financial support is crucial. The American Foundation for Genetic and Nutritional Anthropology is a nonprofit organization with many ongoing research projects exploring the benefits of an instinctive pre-Paleolithic diet such as Genefit Nutrition. Should you consider giving AFGNA your financial support, please contact us for details. Or, you can simply contribute by sending your donations directly to:

> American Foundation for Genetic
>   and Nutritional Anthropology
> P.O. Box 1613
> Hollywood, CA 90078

Your help will be greatly appreciated.

For more information about donations, contact us at donations@afgna.org.

General information about AFGNA is available at http://www.afgna.org.

Fit for Life

APPLYING GENEFIT NUTRITION all the time is not always easy. Social life, business lunches, food supply issues, psychological challenges might often get in the way. Culinary art has been around for quite a while, so don't worry if your way back to a truly natural way of eating looks more like climbing Mount Everest than driving on an empty highway. You may switch back and forth many times until Genefit Nutrition becomes second nature. Always remember that the problem isn't you, but the context we live in. Thousands of years of culinary history can't be wiped out overnight: be patient and take it easy on yourself. But, after all the cleansing and benefits of a Genefit Nutrition 21-day program, it would be a waste to go back to past unhealthy eating habits. If for whatever reason a long-term application can't be part of your life, you will still be looking for a healthy alternative. Among all the options available today one approach to nutrition particularly stands out as a reference. Sixteen years ago, Harvey and Marilyn Diamond made history with their best-selling book *Fit for Life*. Together, they brought pioneer nutritional research into the homes of millions of people. The book sold at eleven million copies worldwide and has been translated into thirty-two languages. But success did not keep Harvey Diamond from raising the bar a step higher by constantly updating his ongoing research, to which he has dedicated the past thirty years of his life. The results of his latest research can be found in his new book *The Fit for Life Solution*, in which he underlines the importance of prevention, periodic mono-dieting, the role of the lymphatic system in the elimination of toxins, and the use of whole, raw foods for better health. Although we do not endorse the use of supplements of any kind, we recommend *Fit for Life* during times Genefit Nutrition can't be applied. In his books Harvey Diamond offers a wide range of easy-to-apply nutritional guidelines, and *Fit for Life* is without doubt an excellent alternative.

More extensive information about Harvey Diamond is available at:

VP Nutrition
P.O. Box 188
Osprey, FL 34229
PHONE: Toll Free 877-335-1509
EMAIL: info@vpnutrition.com
WEB: http://www.vpnutrition.com